THE DANCE CURE

The surprising science to being smarter, stronger, happier

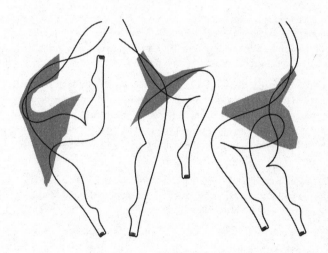

DR. PETER LOVATT

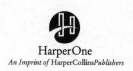

HarperOne
An Imprint of HarperCollins Publishers

THE DANCE CURE. Copyright © 2021 by Peter Lovatt. All rights reserved. Printed in the United States of America. No part of this book may be used or reproduced in any manner whatsoever without written permission except in the case of brief quotations embodied in critical articles and reviews. For information, address HarperCollins Publishers, 195 Broadway, New York, NY 10007.

HarperCollins books may be purchased for educational, business, or sales promotional use. For information, please email the Special Markets Department at SPsales@harpercollins.com.

Originally published as *The Dance Cure* in the UK in 2020 by Short Books.

First HarperOne hardcover published 2021

Interior illustrations © Helena Sutcliffe

FIRST EDITION

Library of Congress Cataloging-in-Publication Data has been applied for.

ISBN 978-0-06-304688-7

21 22 23 24 25   LSC   10 9 8 7 6 5 4 3 2 1

To my mother, for giving me the gift of dance.

To my wife, Lindsey, for dancing with me every day.

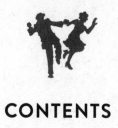

CONTENTS

INTRODUCTION

We are born to dance. Dancing changes the way we feel and think and boosts our self-esteem. We communicate through dance: just as the way we move is influenced by our emotions so we can recognize a person's emotional state from the way they move their body. What's more, our own subconscious movements are influenced by our hormonal and genetic make-up. So dancing brings together our body, our mind and our hormones—no wonder it is such a powerful activity that can make us feel fabulous.

In this book I'm going to take you on an adventure as I explore our urge and desire to dance. It's a story older than civilization, one that predates language, and which set the rules of human societies before the

1

birth of organized religion. A story packed with conflict, jealousy and forbidden love.

As a dance psychologist and teacher, I have witnessed the way dancing has changed the lives of hundreds of people. Some years ago, a woman in her late thirties used to come to my dance classes. Each week she would arrive ten minutes before the class began and I would ask her the normal "new student" questions: Had she danced previously? Did she have any injuries? And each week she would have to remind me that she wasn't a new student, that she had been the previous week . . . and we would both nervously laugh. This happened four weeks in a row—much to my embarrassment—until I finally understood what was going on.

The studio I taught in had a mirror. And, on that fourth week, I used the mirror to teach part of the session. As I scanned the room in the reflection, my eyes alighted on a woman I didn't recognize, whom I must have missed at the beginning of the class. And then, when I turned to face the students, and everyone stopped dancing, I recognized her: it was the woman I kept forgetting. As I watched her make her way to the changing rooms, it suddenly became clear—there was a complete disconnect between this woman's persona off and on stage. On arrival at the class, she looked anxious, tired and worn down and walked with an awkward, heavy gait. But when she danced, she came alive. Her eyes were bright, and she appeared taller and more relaxed. She moved with light-footed steps, and her arms flowed. When she danced, she surrendered herself to joy.

Virginia Woolf, not a person one would necessarily associate with wild and free-spirited dancing, describes this power beautifully. Lying in bed on a winter evening, the 21-year-old Virginia writes of being pulled to her window by the sound of music and laughter from a party across the street: "Dance music . . . stirs some barbaric instinct—you forget centuries of civilization in a second, & yield to that strange passion which sends you madly whirling round the room. . . . It is as though some swift current of water swept you along with it."

I have seen this transformative power in both men and women, old and young. I have seen it in people who have danced for many years, and I have seen it in people for whom dance is a new experience. I have even seen it in businessmen who have previously told me that they don't and indeed cannot dance. And it has nothing to do with how good a dancer someone is, nor is it about any particular style of dance. I have seen it in people when they have been dancing freestyle in nightclubs or performing ballet and other classical forms such as Indian dance; I have seen it in modern forms such as jazz, tap and contemporary dance, in couple dancing such as ballroom and Latin, and in social forms such as line dancing. What all these forms have in common is that they require a particular kind of communication between the brain and the body—using movements that can connect people with themselves and connect them with others.

A special sort of beauty is perceivable in people when they dance. I don't mean beauty in a physical sense. The beauty that is visible through dance has nothing to do with the size or shape of your body. It's about the kind of beauty you show when you are happy, worry-free and living in the moment. Dance plugs people into the here and now. A ballet teacher of mine once said that "dance is movement, and movement is life." Dancing brings the life essence of a person to the fore.

In my case, dance has been transformative in an eminently practical way too. In chapter 1, I will explain how, from being a professional dancer with no academic qualifications, I became a scientist researching at Cambridge University—and how I got there through dance. Indeed, it was largely thanks to dancing that, at the relatively late age of 23, I learned to read.

A huge amount of research has been done on dance in the fields of neuroscience, cognition, biology, medicine, anthropology and evolutionary theory, and the evidence is clear: it shows that the act of dancing brings about specific psychological and physical changes that can play an important role in our lives.

In this book I will describe how dancing affects both our mental processing—i.e., what and how we think—and our emotions. Dancing can reduce anxiety, partly by getting us to focus on the self and live in the moment. Physically, it enables us to control tension and relaxation in key areas of our body, causing us to move with a different purpose from, say, when we walk to get from A to B, or run for exercise. I will explain how our psychological and physical states are intimately related, and how making a change to one of them will lead to a change in the other.

Having explained the science, I will show you a whole range of practical ways in which you can use dance to improve your life. Using laboratory-based evidence, I have created a unique set of combos and dance routines tailored to produce particular effects and emotional changes. The way we move our body affects us at many different levels. Some combinations of movement can calm us and improve our mood; some can make us feel energized and focused; some can help us to think more creatively and speed up our problem-solving ability; still others can make us feel more robust and confident. What's more, these changes are evident to the people around us.

Dance is one of the most powerful forms of communication that we have. It changed my life. And it can change your life, too.

CHAPTER 1

MY STORY

When I dance, I feel different, in lots of ways; I am more aware of my emotions, I find it easier to relate to people, my mind feels less cluttered and, perhaps most importantly, I feel more "me." When I'm moving, listening to music, feeling the groove, jumping, turning, bouncing and preparing to do a double pirouette, I have a feeling of completeness. The world looks, sounds and feels different. My lungs and heart fill up on an expansive breath, and I float, fly and feel completely free.

I also think best when I'm moving. Sitting still never came naturally to me. I fidget, twitch and get distracted by sounds, lights, smells and the feeling of clothes on my body. When my body is still, my mind races from one thought to another, turning at tangents. Moving gives my thoughts an order and a shape—also, interestingly, different types of dance seem to arrange my thoughts in different ways.

As someone who hates sitting down, I hated school. I hated school for other reasons too: I found the lessons difficult—I really struggled to learn the basics of reading and writing; and I didn't fit in. That said, I was also enormously lucky that my secondary school had a dance group. It was called Color Supplement because all the dancers had to wear different-colored Lycra catsuits. Mine was maroon. Perhaps this was the reason very few boys joined Color Supplement— most of the time I was the only one. While all the other boys in my year group were getting changed for soccer, I'd be squeezing myself into a series of Lycra tubes and putting on jazz shoes.

What I found natural, other people found grossly unnatural. And in the late 1970s people weren't shy about coming forward to share what they thought of you. My classmates were no exception. I was called queer, poof, gay-boy, bender, faggot, any name negatively associated with homosexuality at the time. Those words were shouted at me, "Oi, queer, where's your tutu?" and written on blackboards. The unimaginative insults coincided with the onset of puberty and only stopped when I confronted one particularly nasty bully called Ian, who had made it his mission to keep me firmly at the top of the public shaming league.

One day, after a pair of ballet shoes had been discovered in my school bag, Ian moved in for the ultimate humiliation. I was told that he wanted to meet me at the top of the school field, which could only mean one thing. This was where boys fought over girls, honor, social rank, and now, for the first time at my school, ballet shoes. I couldn't refuse. I walked the length of the field and attracted a band of people who followed me. It was all very *West Side Story*. Everyone was laughing excitedly in anticipation of seeing Lycra Boy get beaten up. Ian made the first move; he rushed over and jumped on me. But I was used to having girls sitting on my shoulder, so I was able to hold his weight and, eventually, to push him off. And then, because I wasn't used to letting people drop to the ground, I instinctively tried to grab him as he fell, and he ended up in a makeshift headlock, with his head sticking out from under my arm. I had never punched anyone before, I had never even wanted to punch anyone, but this was far too good an opportunity to pass up. I managed to punch him once for every year he had made my life a misery. Four solid punches landed squarely on his nose with resounding thuds. We broke apart and stared at each other in silence. After a few minutes, as a globule of blood from his nose turned into a torrent, he turned and walked away. All was quiet until a boy in the crowd shouted after him, "Who's the poof now, Ian?" and everyone laughed. This was a turning point for me at school—not only was I free to bring every variety of dance shoe in, it also showed me how much dancing had made me physically stronger. All the push-ups, physical exercises and partner work had made me muscular. Ian and his gang never bothered me again.

As I look back on this, I am relieved that I didn't succumb to the pressure to stop dancing. I'm sure it would have been easier to swap ballet shoes for soccer cleats, but I cannot imagine how empty my life would have been then. I feel sad for all those boys who stop dancing shortly after the onset of puberty. Social pressure is a big part of the problem, but it's not just the throwaway insults that stop boys and men from dancing. Social pressure can come from peers, friends and family, as well as the dance world itself, which can be an uninviting place if you're male. Dance shops are often pink, feminine and child-focused, with many doubling as fancy-dress shops. Dance classes are often taught by women and are full of girls and can therefore be intimidating for boys and men.

The other main reason I hated school was the constant requirement to read and write, which I just couldn't do. I grew up in the 1970s, when dyslexia was not as widely recognized as it is today; and as a slow reader I was labeled "backward" and generally considered to be "a bit thick."

At school I could read the words "dog" and "cat," and I could understand the sentence "the cat sat on the mat." But there were many words I didn't know how to say out loud and words I simply had no idea how to spell, such as "rhythm." I still struggle to select the right spelling for two words that have similar sounds. Imagine hearing the following sentence and having to write it down: "I didn't choose to lose my shoes." I'd hear that the three key words "choose," "lose" and "shoes" rhymed and I'd therefore expect them to have similar spelling rules, but I would soon be in a cold sweat as I would know, deep down, that they didn't. My mind would race around the possibilities, trying to resolve the ambiguity, by which point (buy witch point?) I would have lost the meaning of the sentence altogether.

My struggle to learn the infuriating rules of reading

and writing had a subsequent effect on almost everything else at school. After all, the education we receive at school is based on a learning system that relies on extensive reading. For example, to learn about history we had to read about it in textbooks, and to demonstrate how much we knew about the industrial revolution we had to write everything down. I would always dread that moment in class when the teacher would say, "Open your books at page 230 and read to the end of the chapter." I'd never get to the end of the chapter. I knew it would be pointless trying, so I'd drift off into my own world, stare out of the window, fidget, look around and, inevitably, get told off for distracting other people.

My lack of engagement in the classroom was seen as disobedience, and the group of troublemakers I ended up befriending didn't help. These were students who also struggled with reading. Finding lessons boring, they, like me, were looking elsewhere for stimulation. As our acts of rebellion became ever more elaborate, so too did our punishments, which went from detentions to canings (three strikes each time) and finally a period of suspension from school. Several of us were suspended for moving a teacher's car and sticking apple cores up its exhaust pipe—I did enjoy that day at school! Eventually, some of these friends found themselves on the wrong side of the law, and a few even spent time in police custody and prison. I was lucky; dancing saved me.

However, needless to say, I left school without any written qualifications. While I wasn't put in for exams such as history or geography, I did have to sit for them in English, which I failed spectacularly and repeatedly. As a 16-year-old, I would never have guessed that one day I'd walk into a famous publishing house in Bloomsbury, a fashionable district in the West End of London famous for being home to a host of inspirational English writers, philosophers and artists, and talk about a book I'd written. At 16 I was functionally illiterate. I'd never read a book, and I found it almost impossible to comprehend complex patterns of written words.

After school, I went on to study theatre and creative arts at the local college for two years, which I loved. I then studied dance and musical theatre for another three years at GSA, the prestigious Guildford School of Acting, famous at the time for having a graduate in every single West End musical. Those five years of training were fabulous. Every day was filled, from morning till evening, with classes in dance (ballet, tap, jazz, character, pas de deux, national, contemporary), voice, singing and acting, with the chance to perform in several dance or musical theatre shows every year.

In my second year at GSA, there was just one class with which I struggled, called "Presentation." Every week we were given a theme, or the name of a famous musical theatre lyricist. We'd have to learn a song in that theme or by that lyricist, choreograph it, stage it, find props and costumes and perform the piece the following week in front of the heads of dance, music, voice and acting. It was terrifying. I loved the performing element of this exercise but wasn't so fond of the critique afterwards. The teachers didn't hold back; they were brutal, opinionated and blunt. Motivated by a desire for us to be the very best musical theatre performers and with no time to waste on beating around the bush, they seldom told us what we'd done right and focused instead on telling us exactly what needed to be changed and improved upon. The better you were, the more specific and detailed the notes. Sometimes it's difficult to hold on to a core belief in your own abilities when you face a torrent of "corrections," but that is what we had to do.

I was very lucky to work as a professional dancer for several years. My first job out of GSA was with a variety show that toured throughout England and Scotland, playing at some of the biggest regional theatres, including the Nottingham Theatre Royal, the Birmingham Hippodrome and the Sunderland Empire. I learned a lot about performing for live audiences on that tour, about riding the wave of energy you get from an audience of 1500; and also about trying to give the same performance, with only eighteen people sitting at the back of an otherwise empty auditorium on a sunny Wednesday afternoon.

It was far easier to play to the 1500, especially when it came to the encores. Our variety show had a live band, a big chorus and three principal singers. But for this type of touring show, it was normal to have a soundtrack, or a click track, running in the background throughout the entire show, right up until the final encore, to give the music a fuller, orchestral sound. Our voices were also on the soundtrack, so that when we got completely out of breath towards the end of a big song-and-dance number, we could still be heard clearly throughout the auditorium. This meant the whole show, even the six encores, had to be played out in full once the soundtrack had started. This worked well when we performed to big full houses, but when we played to a virtually empty building at the Lakeside Country Club, where the only people in the audience were my old landlady from Guildford and her bemused husband and daughter, it was difficult to keep the grateful smiles on our faces as we started encore number six. If they hadn't known me, and turned up to show their support, I'm sure they would have left at the intermission and we could all have had an early night.

One of my later dancing jobs was on board the MV *Oceanos* cruiser, as one of four dancers on a six-month contract performing a variety of shows seven nights a week on over a dozen two-week circuits around the Caribbean islands.

I had originally been offered an Equity contract by a prolific musical theatre choreographer to appear in a traditional Christmas pantomime at the Liverpool Empire. "Pantos" are song-and-dance spectaculars with jokes and slapstick humor. But when this fell through, the choreographer's office presented me with the job on the cruise ship. I was thrilled to bits and assumed that the contract would be sound. I should have heeded the saying "When you 'assume' you make an 'ass' out of 'u' and 'me.'" Well, this contract certainly made an ass out of me.

A few months into the job, I got wind that my wages were not being deposited, as I assumed, into my bank account. But when I asked if I could leave the ship, I was told that wasn't an option and that if

I broke the contract, I'd have to pay not only for my own flight back to the UK, but also for a replacement dancer to be flown out to the Caribbean and for their two weeks of rehearsal time, which, needless to say, I couldn't afford. My only way out, I felt at the time, was to behave so atrociously that they would kick me off the ship. Which they did, unceremoniously, leaving me and a fellow dancer stranded 3000 miles from home. Fortunately, my parents came to my aid. Despite not having a lot of money, they wired what they could so that I could fly home.

When I got back to London, I was advised to sue the company to recover the money I was owed. When I wrote to the choreographer asking for my money, he replied that he didn't owe me any money, and he ended his letter with "PS—the correct spelling is 'Caribbean.'" All those useless feelings from school came rushing back to me. The letter I had written was obviously full of spelling errors and incomprehensible grammar. I didn't understand how someone who so obviously owed me money could be so condescending as to sign off by correcting my spelling.

It turned out that the contract I had signed was not provided by Equity, so Equity couldn't help me. (Equity is the performers' union, and among other things, it protects performers from being treated badly by employers.) I was pushed from pillar to post, and it was unclear in which jurisdiction I should pursue a claim. Eventually I let the money go, but the experience made me recognize a need for change in my life. I didn't like the feeling that I could be cheated so easily and realized my reading difficulties were part of the problem.

I spent the summer working to repay my landlady and to get back on an even financial keel. It was during this time that I met a group of very bookish people studying at prestigious universities. The group was made up of girls and boys who were articulate, well-read, worldly wise and, most of all, supremely confident. They gave the impression that they could do anything they set their minds to. And they had a profound effect on my life.

Frank was the alpha male of the group. He'd been head boy at a famous private school and was studying literature at Oxford University when I met him. His parents were wealthy in a way I couldn't comprehend, and his life was the polar opposite of mine. Even though Frank knew about world affairs, politics and fine art, and had a school bag full of qualifications,

I enjoyed and felt comfortable in his company. I had my successes in dance and performing arts, and he had his as a by-product of a traditional education. We both had our distinct talents—until Frank crossed over into my world. Back at Oxford, he put on a production of Mike Leigh's *Abigail's Party* and invited me to the performance in his college. I went along, expecting it to be rubbish. But of course, it wasn't. He'd done a really good job. I left Oxford the next day feeling cross, cheated and humiliated. I'd felt that I was Frank's opposite but equal. Yet his directorial achievement threw everything out of balance.

This thought stayed with me for weeks, buzzing around in my head. It seemed to me that the only real difference between Frank's group of bookish friends and me was that they spent their lives studying books and words and I didn't; I couldn't. I felt I was missing out on great conversations on subjects I knew nothing about because I wasn't reading. I had two choices: I could either carry on being the person who had failed with words, or I could learn to overcome my shortcomings.

I warmed myself up for a reading marathon by reading *The Cross and the Switchblade* by David Wilkerson. I chose that book because one of the girls in the group had just read it in a couple of days. I decided to approach reading as though I were learning a new dance. I knew that I wouldn't understand every sentence, or even every word, but I thought if I could find a rhythm, or sets of different rhythms, within the story, then I could break it down and learn it "one eight at a time." What I also knew from being a dancer was that perfection comes from relentless hours of practice, and success comes in incremental steps. Dancing is multi-layered, and it is possible to learn a new dance one layer at a time. To do this, a dance teacher or choreographer would first give us the feel of the piece by laying out the context: perhaps we might be dancing a scene from *Romeo and Juliet* and had to represent a forbidden desire. Then we would be told the basic structure: that it was to be a pas de deux, a dance for two people. We would look at the types of movements: the lifts and shapes, and how much space we'd be using in the studio. We would discuss who the piece was for, what the audience might expect; we might listen to the music and think about the mood of the piece. Only then would we create or learn some choreography, the actual sequence of movements—but we'd start small, by just learning the feet before adding the arms. All this is what is meant by learning a dance "one eight at a time."

So I started to read. Whenever there was a word that I didn't know how to say, I simply made up a sound for it. There was no one to tell me off if I read "yacht" as anything other than a word that rhymed with "got." The closest I came was to put a "y" sound in front of "act" to make "y-act." I still can't see the logic of how to sound out "-acht." I felt that if the arrangements of letters in words could be arbitrary, then the sound in my head could be arbitrary too. Whenever there was a long sentence with multiple clauses, I simply broke it down, as I would a dance routine, and rather than getting lost in multiple interpretations, I would settle on one and try to ignore the others unless my interpretation became obviously wrong. All this took a very long time.

Many years later, when I was working as a dance psychologist, I carried out an experiment to see how non-dancers process contemporary dance, and I noticed a similarity between how they struggled to make sense of it and how I struggled to process strings of words. The experiment was a "think-aloud protocol" in which participants are asked to say whatever comes into their mind while they are doing a task, in this case watching a piece of dance. People would talk, and I would record their stream of consciousness as they spoke. I found that some people would simply describe what they saw as if they were watching a series of meaningless shapes. Some would speak about the differences between their own abilities and those of the dancers; some would try to make sense of what they were watching by creating a narrative, but when the movements didn't conform to that narrative, they would change the story. Once the participants had tried out several potential narratives that didn't work, they would sometimes give up and say they had no clue what was going on in the piece. What was clear was that there was no "one way" or even a "right way" to read dance, and non-dancers struggle just as much with comprehending movement sequences as poor readers struggle with comprehending sequences of words.

By late autumn, the beginning of the pantomime season, I knew things were changing. Starting to read had given me greater confidence and changed the way that I looked at the world. I had always taken dancing for granted. I thought it was easy. Someone would show me a series of dance moves and I'd remember them. My body seemed to hold a memory for movement patterns, and I could morph from one shape to another naturally. I began to see dancing differently. I realized that dancers can do something extraordinary: learning movement patterns by rote and remembering long sequences of movements is no minor feat. It also occurred to me that the mental requirement for dancing is far more taxing than for other performing arts.

Dancers must learn thousands of subtle changes in body position simply by watching someone demonstrating those movements. They don't write the moves down, and they're not given a book with everyone's moves written out. Imagine if actors or musicians had to learn their parts by heart in this way. When dancers go home at the end of rehearsals, they must practice, but they don't have anything to remind them of the dance moves, other than the music and their own fantastic memory.

Once I realized I was capable of learning and understanding thousands of hours of intricate movement patterns over my life as a professional dancer, I knew I should be able to apply that ability to learning information presented in a written-word form, and thereby learn about current affairs, literature and science. I just needed a route in, and the route in was dance. When the pantomime season finished at the end of January, I left my life in London and, with no qualifications, except for a CSE Grade 1 in Drama (Certificate of Secondary Education; Grade 1 was the lowest level of attainment for a 16-year-old school-leaver) and a diploma from the Guildford School of Acting, I set out on a new path. Sometimes when you need to make a life-changing decision you have to alter your day-to-day habits and move to a new environment. I bought a ticket to Canada and took the train from Montreal to Vancouver. For 3000 miles I read poetry. Feeling the rocking motion of the train created a physical connection with the words on the page. The rhythm and rumble became a soundtrack that transformed words into lyrics. Hearing myself reading was like listening to self-generated rap, and this compelled me to move, making words addictive. I still find it almost impossible to sit still when I read Walt Whitman's "O Captain! My Captain!" It demands movement, and sometimes even a double hand clap at the end of the second line: "O Captain! my Captain! our fearful trip is done, the ship has weather'd every rack, the prize we sought is won [clap-clap]."

Going past herds of nodding donkeys, and through the Rocky Mountains, I learned that once you physically move with information it has a different texture; like walking over sand, stones or grass. You discover new qualities in the ground once you feel it under your feet, rather than simply look at its surface—and I find words to be the same. Lying still on the page they all seem rather bland, but when I move with them our relationship changes; I feel them from a different perspective, and while some give me the same pleasure as lying on a freshly cut lawn, others challenge me to keep my balance, as when I'm walking over a rocky beach. This train journey taught me how to dance with words.

Some months later, I bought a copy of *Anna Karenina* by Tolstoy. (An English translation, of course.) While reading it I fell in love for the first time with a character I had only known through the written word. I fell in love with Kitty. I couldn't stop reading about her. I worried about her when the book was closed; I felt the excitement of anticipating her appearance on the next page; I felt jealous of Levin, her husband, and an aching sense of hopelessness in my unrequited love. There was absolutely nothing I could do to make Kitty notice me. I finished broken-hearted, a changed person. I read *Resurrection* and then moved on to Turgenev and Dostoevsky. Thirty-plus years on, I still have my copy of *Great Short Works of Fyodor Dostoevsky*, pre-owned and inscribed by a Harvard University student called Kelly. That simple inscription became another signpost, and it bolstered my belief that these books would eventually lead me to the illustrious spires of Oxbridge, where I would one day earn my elbow-patched corduroy jacket. I was like an oceangoing liner; once I'd started, I just kept cruising, moving slowly from one great book to another.

In the real world, getting into university was harder than I thought it would be. I decided to study psychology. I thought that I could combine it with drama and dance and perhaps train as a drama or dance therapist and use the creative arts to help people. I bought and read books by Freud and Jung, and I read case studies, such as *Dibs in Search of Self*, *Cry Hard and Swim* and *The Man Who Mistook His Wife for a Hat*. But none of these books offered explanations to the questions I had about the subject. At the same time, I started to contact psychology departments at a couple of universities to ask if they'd let me on to their course. I had no idea how to go about applying to university, but I was told that I would need at least one A-level (an advanced-level subject-specific qualification, normally taken by 18-year-old school-leavers) to do so.

I enrolled in an evening class to study for an A-level in Psychology. To do this, I had to give up working as a professional dancer as I had to be based in one place for a year and I wasn't able to work in the evenings. I attended classes twice a week while I made formal applications for a place at university, and in between I took odd jobs as a delivery driver. Everything was fine; it was all going according to plan. And then, over a period of several weeks in winter, I was rejected by all five of the universities I had applied to. This came as a blow. A hard one. Manchester, Sheffield, University College London, Bristol and Durham all said no. By the time the fifth rejection arrived, I was ready to run. I stopped attending the evening classes and wondered what on earth I'd done: I'd given up a career as a dancer, the only thing I was good at, the only thing that felt natural to me, to go to university—and I hadn't got a place.

During this time, I started dating a girl called Lindsey, whom I'd met at the evening class. She, too, was going through a career change and needed her A-level in Psychology to go to university. She'd been accepted by the university of her choice and was sailing through the course. I'd missed more than half of it, but Lindsey, after much cajoling, managed to persuade me to return for the last few classes of the year and sit the exam. We studied together every night for a month. It was the best thing I could have done, for two reasons: firstly, I sat the exam, and passed—only just, but it was enough to keep me in the academic game; and secondly, I married Lindsey a few months later, and she's been my life partner ever since.

I now took a more strategic approach to getting a university place. I went to visit several university psychology departments and met with various admissions tutors. Fortunately, one of the colleges made me an unconditional offer, and I started my university journey at Froebel College, Roehampton, in September 1990. The grounds of Froebel College were beautiful, and it felt as though I had been picked up and dropped back in time. During my three years there I became fascinated by neurobiology and neuro-psychology, which concern the study of the biological make-up of the brain and what happens to people when the brain is damaged.

At the time, dance and psychology were very sep-arate parts of my life. I learned about psychology in the lab and I danced in the studio, as well as perform-ing in plays and shows—but I knew I didn't want to train as a dance therapist. My parents had worked in a hospital, and I knew this wasn't the environment for me. I wanted something else but didn't know what.

I graduated from Roehampton in 1993 and took up a national scholarship to study for an MSc in Neural Computation at the Center for Cognitive and Computational Neurosciences at the University of Stirling. Neural computation involves building models of the working brain using mathematics and artificial networks. We were a small, odd cohort of students made up of computer scientists, physicists, mathematicians and psychologists, and our aim was to work out how we could build plausible models of the brain and then inflict "brain damage" on them so that we could learn how they recover. It was ambitious. I found the mathematics baffling at first. Lectures would consist of slide after slide of mathematical formulas, composed of what seemed like hundreds of Greek symbols. My evenings were spent learning to distinguish and name the symbols for theta, delta, lambda (which I thought was a drama school). It was a challenging course, and most of the students were super-bright introverts who could absorb pages of mathematical proof in the same way I would learn long dance routines, with no need to write anything down. I struggled with the calculus and algebra but got through in the end and moved on from Stirling to the University of Essex, to take up a scholarship to study for a doctorate in Experimental Cognitive Psychology. Cognitive psychology deals with how humans think, learn, solve problems, use language, perceive the world and remember. Experimental cognitive psychology involves a great deal of laboratory work. I spent three years in a very small lab measuring how much time it took people to read lists of words and afterwards to see which words were the easiest to remember. I was trying to understand how people learn and remember, with an aim to develop appropriate rehabilitation programs for those with brain damage, in particular those with impaired memory and language systems.

When I completed my doctorate, I took up a post-doctoral position in the Research Centre for English and Applied Linguistics in the Faculty of English at Cambridge University. As a dancer I was used to auditioning for jobs where hundreds of hopefuls would be whittled down during successive rounds of dance-offs, but my Cambridge interview was like nothing I had experienced before. A two-day process at one of the oldest, most prestigious universities in the world—which for me was also a magical, end-of-a-rainbow kind of place that I had been dreaming of for the past seven years.

At Cambridge University, I worked as a psychologist on a project to examine how people learn more than one language. I was interested in how people "think" in different languages and how they store and remember words that might have the same or different meanings across different languages; as well as how they read new (foreign) words and make sense of them, and then learn to understand complex linguistic patterns. I also became interested in the relationship between dyslexia and memory. For the first time, I started to read about some of the problems that people with dyslexia have seeing, coding and remembering words. The descriptions I read in the literature could have been written about me and the problems I had with reading: the difficulty of reading "exception" words (that is, words whose sound doesn't match their letters), the difficulty of remembering which words in a very long sentence go together, and the difficulty of focusing on individual words in large blocks of text. Learning about the cognitive models of these reading difficulties helped me to understand why I had found reading so hard and how I had been able to overcome these challenges.

My time at Cambridge University as an academic psychologist marked the end of a long journey. It had taken me ten years, and I now had a BSc, MSc and PhD in psychology. I felt as though I'd reached the summit of Mount Everest. So I did exactly what everyone does once they've reached the summit of a mountain: I turned around and walked back down. After two years I left Cambridge and started to plan how I could combine my expertise in psychology with the subject I loved most in the world, dance. The Dance Psychology Lab was the result.

Seeing people's lives transformed by dance is an awe-inspiring experience. You might say it's magical, but that would be wrong. There is nothing magical, mystical or spiritual about the transformative power of dance, but it has been a mystery, until now. I set up the Dance Psychology Lab so that I could use advanced scientific techniques to study the relationship between movement and the brain, to help me understand why and how dancing is such a powerful human behavior. What I found was extraordinary: people with Parkinson's disease and dementia getting a new lease of life; an increase in the self-esteem of teenagers; reductions in depression and anxiety in adults; increases in social bonding between people; and fundamental changes in the way people think and solve problems. All because of dancing.

The Dance Psychology Lab is my favorite place in the world, because it's where I can collaborate with dancers and scientists to explore scientific ideas, and its dance floor is the springboard from which I can bounce around the world working with multinational corporations, schools and educational establishments and healthcare providers. In the next chapter, I will explain the surprising secrets of dance, and how they can make you smarter, stronger and happier.

CHAPTER 2

A UNIVERSAL LANGUAGE

"Dance. *v. intransitive.* To leap, skip, hop, or glide
with measured steps and rhythmical movements of
the body, usually to the accompaniment of music,
either by oneself, or with a partner or in a set."
—*The Oxford English Dictionary*

For someone who has spent their whole life dancing, the question "What is dance?" *should* be
simple to answer. I know dancing when I see it, and I
certainly feel it when I'm doing it, but defining what
is, and what is not, dance is a much more difficult
question to answer than you might think. Where
does movement stop, and dance begin?

If someone is not performing any of the actions

listed in the *OED* definition, can we say that they are definitely not dancing? I don't think so. I often dance without a leap, skip, hop or glide; sometimes I dance without a measured step, and sometimes I'm not the least bit rhythmic. Therefore, I don't think we can rely on this definition as it doesn't allow for the full breadth of what dancing is and how to distinguish it from not-dance.

I much prefer this description by Jacques d'Amboise, the famous American dancer and choreographer: "Dance is your pulse, your heartbeat, your breathing. It's the rhythm of your life. It's the expression in time and movement, in happiness, joy, sadness and envy."

I love that. Dance is the expression of emotion in movement—which also makes it a communal thing, arguably one of the most socially powerful and communicative activities there is. And that is what we are going to examine in this first part of this book: how dancing forms the basis of the most highly sophisticated language system we have, and how rhythms and shared movements bring us together, helping to build relationships and mutual trust. If you thought words were powerful, just wait until you see what movement can do.

RHYTHM

OK, here we go, & 5, 6, 7, 8! What I've always loved about disco music from the 1970s and 1980s is the hypnotic beat of the 4/4 rhythm:

1, 2, 3, 4,
1, 2, 3, 4,
1, 2, 3, 4,
1, 2, 3, 4 . . .

Listening to Donna Summer singing "I Feel Love" for eight minutes straight sends me into a trance. Framed within a four-beat rhythm, there is layer upon layer of changing color that empties your brain of all thoughts; just like the endorphin high of a long-distance runner carried along by the repetitive monotony of their steps. I get the same sensation from a steady beat. I feel as though the music is a puppeteer and all my movements are involuntary. If you don't know what I'm talking about, try it, and take some time to practice; it produces a feeling of awe and wonder. Search for the original 12" record from 1977. You don't have to do anything clever: just close your eyes and focus on the music—headphones might help. If you feel an urge to move, keep that movement small; if you need a starter, tap your foot or finger or nod your head. Keep it anchored on the strong regular beat—1, 2, 3, 4—and keep going until you're not thinking about what you're doing. Don't let self-consciousness destroy your groove. Lose yourself. Now let your mind go deeper into the rhythm. You and the music. By keeping the movements discrete, you can do this form of dancing sitting at a desk, on the bus, even walking down the street. Another disco tune that you could practice to is "Cuba" by the Gibson Brothers—listen out for the syncopated hand clapping (clapping on an off-beat—very popular in the 1970s) about halfway through. It builds during the final 90 seconds, so stay with it. Then, of course, there's always Michael Jackson, who cuts up a standard 4/4 beautifully in "Wanna Be Startin' Somethin'."

The drive to seek out rhythmic patterns in our environment and respond to them physically is natural for humans. And it begins very early on. A team of scientists from Holland and Hungary discovered in a neonatal-neuroscience experiment that two-day-old babies can recognize and remember auditory rhythms.[1] The babies were fitted with caps with electrodes on the inside to measure the electrical activity going on in their brains as drum-and-bass music was played to them, even when they were asleep. The human brain is active all the time, and it's constantly responding to what's happening both in our body and around us. Some people believe that we only use about 10% of our brain at any time, but that isn't true. The neurons in our brain fire constantly: it's like a New Year's Eve fireworks display erupting in our heads 24 hours a day, 365 days of the year. It is this that the scientists were able to measure in the babies: every flash, bang, oo and ahh.

The scientists then played the same music again but this time took out some of the beats. The question was, would the babies notice that some of the beats were missing? Well, the babies' brains reacted differently when they heard the section of music that contained the missing beat, and this convinced the scientists that babies as young as two days old could recognize and remember rhythmic patterns. This suggests that the capability to detect a beat in rhythmic sound is something we are born with.

Perception of rhythm is just the first part of unlocking the magic of Donna Summer's "I Feel Love." The desire, urge or need to move in response to the music comes from a brain process called "sensorimotor coupling," whereby a sound triggers the parts of the brain responsible for movement, either giving us an urge to move or actually making us move. The movements of different parts of our body are controlled by different parts of the brain. The same process occurs with the startle reflex, when we hear a sudden, unexpected noise that makes us jump.

One of my favorite university studies into the urge to dance was carried out in California.[2] Scientists wanted to find out which piece of music was most likely to activate the sensorimotor area of the brain. Before you read on, can you guess which genre of music—folk, rock, jazz or R&B/soul—is most likely to make people want to move? And which particular song?

To find out, scientists played 148 excerpts from these genres and asked people to say how much each piece gave them an urge to move. What they found was that R&B/soul music was rated as groovier than folk, rock and jazz and that, in general, fast music was rated as groovier than slow music. The grooviest piece of music was "Superstition," a track released by Stevie Wonder in 1972, a funky-soul classic.

Another piece of music that produces a strong urge to move for me is a 1962 tune by Quincy Jones called "Soul Bossa Nova." Have a listen and I challenge you to keep still!

SYNCHRONICITY: HOW DANCING HELPS US COMMUNICATE

When we combine an innate perception of rhythm with a biologically determined impulse to move, we can understand why people start to move together when they hear the same rhythms, and how, in turn, that shared movement will create its own sounds and rhythms, which will again feed back and become a stimulus that everyone will respond to. Children's play is often highly synchronized; for example, they love games that involve clapping, or running and chasing, or holding hands and skipping together. Clapping games, where groups of people chant rhythms and make percussive noises by clapping hands with each other, and against their bodies, are centuries old. The pat-a-cake, pat-a-cake game dates back to 1698. The behavior of very young children may be driven by a specific human motivation to synchronize movements with other people during shared rhythmic activities, and this extends to a liking for listening and moving to music. Moving together can unite people socially and have a positive effect on their willingness to help each other.

Humans are not unique in moving to a groove. If

you have not yet seen Snowball the Cockatoo dancing to "Everybody" by the Backstreet Boys on YouTube, look it up. For some creatures, synchronizing movement with the environment can mean the difference between life and death. For example, it's thought that orangutans move in synchrony with the natural sway of branches when swinging from one tree to another.[3] Being able to synchronize their movements in this way before launching towards a tree is fairly vital for their survival. Any miscalculation and they might come crashing down to the forest floor. Humans have to deal with something like this when getting on and off escalators. The way we synchronize our movements with our environment can have profound consequences for our relationships with other people, the way we think and solve problems, our biological rhythms, and the way we feel.

Dance creates a magnetic force between us, which draws us together. At times, when we dance with someone in a nightclub or at a party, even if there's a distance of several feet between us, it can feel as though there's a physical connection between our body and theirs. George Bernard Shaw described it perfectly when he wrote that dancing is "the perpendicular expression of a horizontal desire legalised by music."

When people move in synchrony, for example,

when they walk or sing together, amazing things happen. If you want a person to like you more, then one of the first things you should do is go for a walk with them, and walk at their pace. Synchronize your walking speed with theirs, and magic happens. I was astonished when I first discovered that this simple act of synchronization leads people to have more positive feelings towards each other. Moving together in time is a form of non-verbal communication that connects us emotionally. Scientists have found that we trust people more when we move in synchrony, and we also feel more affinity with them.[4] I love it when science confirms a popular idea. The saying "Before you judge a man, walk a mile in his shoes" means that before you make a judgment about a person you must empathize with them and understand their experiences, challenges and ideas. Moving together has been proven to facilitate this process. The simplest act is all it takes.

That said, social dancing—dancing at parties and in public—is not to everyone's taste. While for some there is nothing to beat a house party in full swing, for others the very idea will be horrendous. And there's a good reason why. Although dancing is the most natural thing to do, and social dancing has been a fundamental part of human and animal societies for millennia,[5] humans can be extraordinarily self-conscious. They differ from the rest of the animal kingdom through their capacity to judge; they self-monitor in a way that birds and bees don't, and they also make value judgments about themselves.[6] Imagine if a bird was self-conscious of its colorful plumage, or if a bee was afraid to waggle-dance the location of pollen and nectar because it thought the other bees in the hive might think it looked stupid.

Self-consciousness holds us back from doing things that we have a natural urge to do. Often this can be put down to a straightforward fear of embarrassing ourselves or of not being talented enough, but sometimes the beliefs or restrictions of our social environment can also play a part. Some schools of psychotherapy believe this inner conflict is caused by the struggle between our natural desires and the teachings of a particular religion, faith or societal norm. Anyone who has seen the film *Footloose* will remember the story of teenager Ren McCormack, who moves to a small, religious town where all dancing and rock music are banned, branded as "spiritual corruption" by the local authorities. Despite their best efforts, the council cannot constrain the teenagers' desires to dance, and a protest ensues to overturn the law. But for Kevin Bacon, who plays the lead character, the best scene in the film comes when

Ren tries to teach his rhythmically challenged friend Willard to dance: "There's an innocence that's captured there, of just this guy trying to teach this other guy a couple of moves, and I think that's why the movie was popular—more so than any kind of stand-alone dance or gymnastic moves."

Interestingly, Chris Penn—who plays the left-footed Willard in the film—really couldn't dance prior to filming, but the choreographers managed to teach him the routines by relating the dance moves to wrestling, something that he was proficient at!

Fear of dancing due to self-consciousness is a feeling that many of us can relate to. Who hasn't witnessed the scene at a party where some guests are quick to get up and dance, drawn together by the music and shared movement, while others keep themselves separate, glued to the edge of the room by awkwardness and fear? I write more about the second group in chapter 5. For now, let's focus on the lucky people who embrace the natural urge to dance socially.

BUILDING TRUST

Dancing with other people is great for developing relationships and building trust because of the changes it stimulates in our brains. Scientists at Oxford University think that our innate pain-relieving system—otherwise known as the endogenous opioid system—might be working overtime when we dance, and this makes us feel good about the people we are dancing with.[7]

The dancing dons at Oxford tested the relationship between dancing, pain and social bonding and found that they were all linked. Hundreds of people were taught some simple dance moves and then split into two groups, the same-dance group and the different-dance group. The former had to perform the same dance moves at the same time as each other (imagine a group of people all doing the Macarena in perfect unison), while the latter had to do a different set of movements at the same time (imagine three people in a group, one of them doing the Macarena, another person doing the Hokey Pokey, and the third doing the Hustle). Then they measured both groups' pain threshold, by inflating a blood pressure cuff on their arm until the pain became unbearable. Finally, they asked everyone questions about how socially bonded they felt to the people they were dancing with. Here are some of the questions they asked:

- How much do you trust the people you were dancing with?

- How connected do you feel to the people you were dancing with?
- How likable are the people you were dancing with?
- How similar in personality do you feel to the people you were dancing with?

They also asked the participants to look at a series of circles and to pick the one that best represented their relationship with the other dancers (see diagram below).

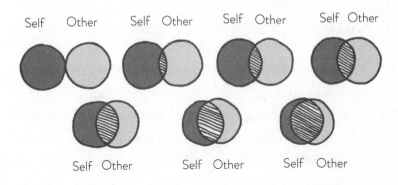

What the researchers found was very surprising. After everyone had danced, there were huge differences between the two groups. Those in the same-dance group felt more socially bonded to the people they had danced with, and could cope with more pain, compared to those in the different-dance group.

Dancing together gives us a natural high because it leads to increased activation of our endogenous opioid system. This makes us feel pleasure, and it changes the way we feel about the people we are dancing with. We trust our dance partners more, we feel more connected to them, we like them more and we think their personality is more similar to ours. We also feel less of a distance between where we end and they begin. It is no wonder that people fall in love when they dance.

DANCING, FERTILITY AND LOVE

While Kevin and his mates spend their Friday nights at the Tap 'n' Tin in Chatham, grooving to the latest urban grime, great crested grebes are doing something similar down at the local lek. The great crested grebe is a type of water bird, and it is famous for its elaborate mating displays. A lek is a group of male animals that come together to engage in competitive mating displays, in the hope of enticing females of the species. There are many similarities between Kevin and his friends, and a flock of great crested grebes.

An animal's mating displays are thought to communicate, or signal, traits that carry information about its quality. The females watch the displays and make a choice about which males to mate with based on the information communicated in them. The movement displays of animals communicate characteristics such as energy and intensity; while the complexity of the movement and the duration of it can be a good indicator of strength and fitness.

According to Charles Darwin, dance plays an important role in the human mate selection process; so when men go to the local nightclub, it is as if they are creating their own human lek. Like birds, humans communicate and signal a great deal when they move and dance, and this might influence their success in finding a mate. But with the absence of feathers, and with no discernible tail to shake, what can humans display about themselves when they're having a wiggle to "Stayin' Alive"?

Well, first off, dancing is physical, and therefore demonstrates a person's vitality, which might be an indicator of their health. We can see how good they are at learning and memory, by the way they pick up sequences of movement patterns; and how attentive they are, by the way they imitate other people's movements. We can see creativity in the way people change or embellish their movements and how well they synchronize their movements to the music and with other people. But we can also see deep into an individual's personality when they cut a rug.

Take the Dr. Dance Terpsichorean Personality Quiz to see how you signal your personality as you dance.

Imagine you're dancing at a party or at a wedding, and answer the following questions:

	Disagree	Neutral	Agree
I am always trying out new dance moves	O	O	O
I pay attention to the correct detail of the dance; it's important to get it right	O	O	O
Everyone notices me when I dance	O	O	O
I dance in the same way as everyone else	O	O	O
I am absolutely terrified to dance	O	O	O

The way you answered these questions will reveal something about your personality. Let's take them one by one.

I am always trying out new dance moves

Your answer to this statement tells us about your openness to new experiences. Trying out new dance moves is a sign that you like to learn new things and that you enjoy new experiences and complexity. This is linked to personality traits such as insightfulness, imagination and spontaneity. If you disagreed with this statement, it suggests you are relatively conventional and perhaps more on the rational than the creative side.

I pay attention to the correct detail of the dance; it's important to get it right

This tells us how conscientious you are. Paying close attention to the details of the dance is a sign that you are dependable and self-disciplined, and of an organized and thorough nature. If you disagreed with this statement, it suggests that you may be somewhat disorganized or careless.

Everyone notices me when I dance

The way you answered this statement tells us how extroverted you are. Dancing in a way that makes everyone notice you is a sign that you are enthusiastic and that you get your energy and drive from other people, and are of an energetic, assertive and talkative nature. If you disagreed with this statement, it suggests you are more reserved and quiet, apt to watch and wait before you leap into things.

I dance in the same way as everyone else

The way you answered this statement tells us how agreeable you are. Dancing in the same way as everyone else is a sign that you are cooperative and friendly, and of a warm and sympathetic nature. If you disagreed with this statement, it suggests that you like going your own way, rather than following the crowd, but also that you tend to be critical and quarrelsome.

I am absolutely terrified to dance

The way you answered this statement tells us how neurotic you are. Being too afraid to dance in public might be a sign that you experience emotional instability and are feeling negative emotions. This could mean you are a person who is anxious and easily upset. If you disagreed with this statement, it suggests that you are calm and emotionally stable.

When we dance, our personality is just as vivid as a set of bright feathers, but dancing also sends signals that are much more deeply rooted than our personality.

Two sets of researchers have recently examined the links between dance and fertility, and their results are intriguing. My research team was one of these groups, but before I reveal what my team found, I want to tell you about the other study, carried out in a lap-dancing club by a team from the University of New Mexico in Albuquerque.[8] Together these studies suggest that women do indeed signal their degree of fertility when they move.

Lap dancing is a type of erotic dance, where women, typically wearing nothing but a G-string, gyrate and dance on the laps of fully dressed men. Men pay a fee to a dancer for a lap dance, and at the end of a given period of time, if the man wants the dance to continue, he can pay the dancer a tip.

The Albuquerque team set out to determine the relationship between the fertility of a small group of lap dancers and the amount they earned in tips across a 60-day period. What they found was that women who were cycling naturally, that is, women who were not using hormonal contraception, earned significantly more tips per shift (US$335 on average) when they were at the fertile stage of their cycle than when they were either at the less fertile, luteal stage (US$260 on average) or while they were menstruating (US$185). It is worth pointing out that those women who were using hormonal contraception earned, across the month, about 30% less than naturally cycling women, and they did not earn the same mid-cycle rise in tips.

These tip patterns suggest that the men were sensitive to the estrus behavior of the lap dancers. It is not absolutely clear why the men gave higher tips, but the researchers think that it may be due to either higher levels of attractiveness during the fertile stage, scent changes, or changes in soft-tissue symmetry. After all, the lap dancers were topless, and their breasts were close enough to the men to be inspected in some detail. One thing that I found interesting about the conclusions drawn by the Albuquerque researchers was that they thought that changes in fertility were not likely to have been communicated through changes in the way the women danced. I wanted to test this out. However, as I thought it would be unlikely that I would be allowed to take my research team into a lap-dancing club to film, I decided to collect data in a different way.

With my research team, I turned our university nightclub into a late-night petri dish. We filmed people dancing in the most naturalistic setting with the hope of being able to answer the following questions: First, if it is the case that women communicate their fertility to men, do they do it through the way they move and dance and do they, therefore, move differently at different stages of their fertility cycle? Second, if so, in what way do they move differently? Third, if they do move differently, do men notice? I set about answering these questions using the films I had made of people dancing and with some sophisticated, state-of-the-art eye-tracking equipment.

I had a comprehensive set of data on all the women I had filmed, and this included information about whether they were using hormonal contraception, whether they had had a period in the last three months, when their last period had started and how long their normal cycle lasted. From this information I was able to use established techniques to estimate whether the dancers were in the fertile, luteal or menstrual-bleeding phase of their cycle. Without telling them that I was examining the relationship between fertility and dance, I asked the researchers to analyze the dancers' moves in detail. They made notes of which parts of the body women moved, how much they moved them, which way they were facing, the variety and frequency with which they changed their movements and how they used the space on the dance floor. Once we had this information, we compared the movement styles of the women at the three different fertility stages, and what we found suggests that women do, indeed, move differently according to how fertile they are.

Women who were at the most fertile stage of their cycle isolated and moved their hips more in relation to their other body parts. When women were at the less fertile stages of their cycle, they still moved their hips, but they moved other body parts—hands, feet and head—just as much. So, just like the peacock showing off his feathers, females like to swing those hips.

I then wanted to see if men would notice these differences in body movement. To measure this, I projected life-sized videos of all the women dancing onto a large screen and fitted the men with eye-tracking devices so that I could record exactly where they were looking as they watched each woman dance. I found that when women isolated a particular body part, that's where men looked. When women moved lots of different body parts, men constantly changed where they looked. Further analysis found that where men looked on the dancers' bodies was also dependent on how fertile the women were. For example, men tended to look more at the hip region of fertile women who were isolating this region more; and they tended to look all over the body of less fertile women who were moving lots of body parts simultaneously.

Finally, I wanted to know how attractive the men found the different women's dancing. It seems that attractiveness is all in the hips. Men rated the hip-moving, fertile women as more attractive than less fertile women, who use less isolation in their body movements.

The implications of these findings go far beyond dancing in nightclubs and mate selection. They are hugely relevant to the way we interact as a society. People make judgments about us based on the way we move, all the time—at work, on the bus, as we walk along the street. And the way we move our body is influenced by our underlying body chemistry.

DANCE AS A TOOL FOR SOCIAL COHESION (AND SUBVERSION)

Flash mobs might be seen as the ultimate in social dancing; they can act as a force for instant community, but are also wonderfully subversive. When you dance in unexpected places, it temporarily changes the environment and people don't know how to respond. It causes a social splash. I've danced in several flash mobs, and the basic elements are always the same. You go to a social space, such as a town center, train station or library, and one person starts to dance, then another person joins in, and then another until it snowballs and lots of people are all doing the same dance routine. It should be as unexpected as a snowstorm on a summer's day. There is an added element of surprise because no one can predict who the next person to join in will be. Before people join in, they pose as unsuspecting passers-by.

My favorite flash mob on YouTube is called "Sound of Music | Central Station Antwerp (Belgium)," and it features over 200 dancers. I love two things about this flash mob: the reaction of the passers-by, their surprise when the music begins, their delighted, smiling expressions and their clapping along; and the comments left by people who have watched the video. They are all so positive and demonstrate the emotional effect that public dancing has. Several people have commented that the routine made them cry because of the joy it exudes; others have said that mass social dancing like this shows the best of humanity. One person wrote: "This is what the world needs more of, more flash mobs and less lynch mobs! Our world is too filled with hate and indifference. I wish we could put love and joy back in our daily lives."

Dance has been used to spread love and joy since the beginning of time. But not everyone is in favor of dancing flash mobs. In some countries, group dancing in public, without permission, breaks several laws, including trespassing and disorderly conduct, and organizers can be prosecuted for not having civil or public liability insurance. In the USA, there is even a lawyer who specializes in flash mob law. The tension between people's desire to dance spontaneously in unregulated environments and a society's need to maintain law and order is seen in lots of forms of dance.

Nowhere was the tension between the police and happy-go-lucky dancers more evident than in the 1980s UK rave culture. Raves were predominantly illegal gatherings of thousands of people in pop-up locations, such as disused warehouses, barns and fields. Rave organizers would turn up with huge sound systems, and people would travel from hundreds of miles away to dance all night long. The police, who were always playing catch-up, would put up roadblocks to stop events getting any bigger, but they were powerless to close a rave down once there was a critical mass of dancing bodies.

But the power of the police to close down a rave changed in 1994, when the British government passed the Criminal Justice and Public Order Act which, among other things, outlawed unlicensed gatherings, such as raves, where amplified music was played. The Conservative government of the time clearly had a problem with two of the most fundamental aspects of what it is to be a human: to come together and to dance. Thousands marched on Westminster in protest.

The way in which people danced at raves was influenced by electronic dance music, such as techno, house and acid, and the speed at which it was played. Typically, rave music was played at an average speed of 120–130 beats per minute (bpm). This is interesting because it's about the same rate at which the heart of a 20-year-old beats when they're engaged in moderately intensive exercise. At this bpm, healthy young ravers can keep dancing for long periods of time.

Rave DJs would control huge crowds of dancers by alternating the rhythm and bpm of the music they played throughout the night. Good DJs were able to bring a crowd close to a frenzied climax by raising the speed of the music to between 160 and 220 bpm and then bringing it down again to a manageable, maintainable 130 bpm. The effect of raising the bpm to 160–220 is that, to keep up with the beat, dancers must be working at close to, or even exceeding, their maximum heart rate (which for 20-year-olds is about 200 bpm).

At this bpm their dance moves become more like spontaneous, automatic, muscular twitches than anything planned or choreographed, and it is at this stage that they are thought to enter into a trance-like state where the body moves as a direct response to the music, so that the sensorimotor coupling of music and movement is more like an automatic startle reflex than a choreographed or planned-in-advance set of movements. A state without time for conscious planning. At this stage, the dancer is completely under the control of the music and, ultimately, the person controlling the music, the DJ. Once in a DJ-induced trance, there is little definition in time, just the constant beat of the music, until sunrise.

When people go into a trance, or a trance-like state, they experience a change in their mindset, a much greater shift than a mere change in mood. A trance resembles a hypnotic state; people become less aware of what's going on around them, and some even say they lose consciousness. Others say it's like being in a semi-conscious daydream, a bit like that time first thing in the morning when you're halfway between being asleep and awake, when your arms and legs don't feel like they belong to you and you can't work out where you are.

People in a trance-like state may experience dizziness or vertigo, accompanied by a sense of disappearance or loss of self and changes in bodily perception. They may begin to experience a perception of collective consciousness. So, in one sense, a trance-like state is an altered state of consciousness, a fundamental change in the conscious mindset.

WHEN GROUP DANCING TIPS OVER INTO TRANSGRESSION

Dancing might not be the first activity that comes to mind when you think of transgression. But in some societies, it is deemed so dangerous that attempts are made to control it for fear that it might corrupt morals. For hundreds of years, people in authority have controlled who can dance, who can interact with dancers, and the type of dancing that people can do. In certain circumstances, dancing has been banned altogether.

Even now in England and Wales, you must have a premises license if you intend to provide a space for people to dance in. Otherwise you can be fined £1000, sent to prison for up to six months, or both. In Sweden, a dance permit was required for public dance events up until 2016, when the Swedish parliament, the Riksdag, very wisely voted unanimously to do away with this law.

In August 2012, seventeen people paid the ultimate price for dancing. They were beheaded by the Taliban for taking part in an activity that is forbidden by Islamic law: dancing in a mixed-gender group. Islamic law does not prohibit dancing per se; in fact, there is a long tradition of dancing in Muslim cultures, but there are certain circumstances where dancing is absolutely *haram* (forbidden). Dancing is seen as abominable wherever alcohol is present, where men and women are gathered together, if the movements are languid or effeminate, and if it is done "to excess." In all other conditions, dancing is fine. For example, Islam permits a woman to dance in front of her husband to please or arouse him, but she mustn't dance in front of other men—or women. The rationale for not dancing in front of other women is that it might lead to unwanted temptation and attraction. One *fatwa* (a ruling on a point of Islamic law), states:

> With regard to dancing on the part of women, it is an evil action and we cannot say that it is permissible, because we have heard of incidents that have occurred among women because of it. If it is done

by men that is even worse, because that is men imitating women, and the evil involved is well known. If dancing is done among a mixed group of men and women, as some of the foolish do, that is even worse because of the mixing and great *fitnah* [temptation] involved, especially when that is done at a wedding party.

Many religious groups have a problem with dancing. Christian sects throughout history have seen it as "the devil's work," and tales of its destructive effects have been recounted as warnings. Dancing, with its implications of physical and mental freedom, does not fit with the solemn strictures of most traditional religions, and any sort of dancing that ventures into a public space and catches a mood, drawing in large numbers of people, can be deemed dangerous. Take the story of a certain Frau Troffea, who, one day in 1518, went down to the riverbank in Strasbourg and began to dance. She danced alone, and no music could be heard. She seemed to be in her own world, moving frenetically to the rhythms in her head for several days. Gradually the townsfolk began to gather around, mesmerized by her performance, and one by one they joined in, until there was a heaving mass dancing on the riverbank, non-stop, day and night. The riverbank became drenched in blood as the dancers' feet blistered and split, and by the time the dancing frenzy was over, some 30 days later, dozens had dropped dead.

No one knows why Frau Troffea started to dance on the riverbank, or what caused hundreds of people to join in with her, but this story is not unique. There are many stories of similar "dancing plagues"[9] in history: the earliest report is from 1017, when an outbreak in eastern Saxony is said to have lasted a whole year and built up to a frenzied climax. A number of possibilities have been posited, including a type of food poisoning known as ergotism, which results from eating ergot, a mold that grows on cereals and causes people to hallucinate and dance in a wild manner. It's also possible that the "plagues" could be an emotional response to a repressive society, triggered by social catastrophe or hardship.

In the sixteenth century, when belief in divine curses and bewitchments was widespread, Frau Troffea's dance plague was attributed to satanic possession. The Christian authorities in Strasbourg decided that the only way to cure her and her fellow dancers was through religious salvation. They loaded groups of dancers on to carts and took them to local churches where priests carried out ceremonies to exorcise the evil spirits.

A few decades later, in 1562, John Knox, the founder of the Presbyterian Church of Scotland, wrote that "the reward of dancers . . . will be to drink in Hell." He wasn't keen on "fiddling and flinging" either. I'm glad I wasn't brought up in Scotland in the sixteenth century; I'm not sure how I would have restrained my urge to dance, particularly had I been listening to a fiddle player. By 1649, the Church of Scotland had banned dancing because it was associated with drunkenness, gluttony, immodesty and lechery—sounds like a typical Saturday night out in most UK towns today. By 1684, distrust of dancing by puritanical Christians had spread across the Atlantic to New England. The Puritan leader Increase Mather was so afraid of how mixed-gender and promiscuous dancing might corrupt society that he wrote a 30-page pamphlet called "An arrow against profane and promiscuous dancing. Drawn out of the quiver of the scriptures." In his fire-and-brimstone sermon, he preached that "the unchaste touches and gesticulations used by dancers have a palpable tendency to that which is evil." The link between dancing and being evil is reinforced several times throughout the text. This must have scared the living daylights out of his audience and made them resist their urge to dance.

That dancing bans have lasted until the present day in some parts of both the Islamic and Christian worlds is perhaps not so surprising. What does seem remarkable, though, is the civil ban on some forms of dancing and movement. While the faith-based bans are rooted in the notion that dancing might lead to immoral behavior, civil bans on dancing are founded on arbitrary decisions and the personal whim of rule makers, rather than on any reason or system. In 2011, a magistrate in Australia told a man that he was too old to dance at a rock concert. Richard Fuller was 43 years of age at the time and had been dancing along energetically, lost in the music of Cold Chisel, his favorite band. He needed more space, so he moved to the aisle of the theatre where he could double fist-pump to his heart's content. Richard never got to dance to the band's anthemic finale, as he was removed from the theatre for dancing in the aisle by the venue's security. In the heat of the moment, Richard Fuller slapped one of the security guards and found himself in court. Ross Mack, the magistrate, fined him $450 for common assault, but more importantly, I think, said in his summing up: "You are too old to dance,

Mr. Fuller." Of course, I agree that Fuller deserved to be fined for slapping a security guard—there is certainly no excuse for that sort of behavior—but to be told this by a civil officer of the law sends the message, firstly, that dancing is only for the young, which is clearly wrong; and secondly, that representatives of local authorities have influence over when, how and which people in a society should move their bodies. Take this idea to its extreme and imagine what life would be like!

CHAPTER 3

DANCING AND
THE BRAIN

I t all begins in our brains. The human brain is special-
ized for the control of movement—it needs to be, in
order to manipulate our 600-plus muscles. The motor
cortex, located at the rear of the frontal lobe, is involved
in the planning, control and execution of voluntary
movements. Meanwhile, the basal ganglia, a set of
structures deep within the brain, work with the motor
cortex to coordinate movements and may in addition
act as a filter to block out unsuitable movements, such
as that ill-advised funky chicken. The cerebellum, at
the back of the skull, also performs several roles, including integrating information from our senses so that our
movements are perfectly fluid and precise.

Just lifting a glass of water to our mouths involves an unimaginably complicated sequence of nerve impulses, so how can our brains cope with a full-blown dance routine? In 2006, researchers at the University of Texas Health Science Center at San Antonio asked amateur tango dancers to perform a basic dance step known as a "box step" while lying in a PET (positron emission tomography) scanner.[10] The way people dance tango in a brain scanner is like this: They lie flat on their backs, their heads kept perfectly still with a thermal-plastic mask, and they have a radioactive substance injected into their bloodstream via a needle in the arm to enable the scientists to measure brain activity. With their knees bent at 90 degrees and wearing socks, they move their feet on a sloped, slippery surface in a kind of tango-esque pattern. They are not allowed to move any other part of their body. In the scans, the researchers saw activation in a region of the brain called the precuneus, which is associated with spatial perception. They believe that this region creates a map of our body's positioning in space, helping us to keep track of our torso and flailing limbs as we plot our path across the dance floor.

Of course, dancing also tends to involve music. Comparing scans of the tango dancers' brains both with and without music, the researchers noticed that those performing to music had more activity in a particular region of the cerebellum called the anterior vermis, which receives input from the spinal cord. It might be that this region of the brain acts as a kind of neurological metronome, coordinating our different brain areas and helping us keep time to the beat.

Dancing stimulates the link between the body and brain. In fact, it provides a full brain and body massage! Signals are relayed from the motor area of the brain to nerves, muscles and joints, and the moving body also sends signals back to different parts of the brain and creates activity both deep down at the core of the nervous system and in the neocortex, the brain's outer layer.

I can remember an hour before taking my driving test in 1982, dancing to "Freebird" by Lynyrd Skynyrd in my parents' sitting room. It is a heavy-rock anthem that builds to an amazing, head-banging, sweaty, exhausting crescendo. As I shook my head and limbs to the music, I collected up the tension from the different parts of my body and released it in an explosion of energy. When I took my driving test, I was on fire: three-point turn, a breeze, emergency brake executed within the space of a postage stamp, and safe stopping distances repeated to perfection. "Freebird" had activated all the areas of my brain that I needed to drive and recognize sets of road signs: spatial awareness, visual perception, sequencing and memory. Dancing around my parents' sitting room had woken up my mind and helped me pass my driving test.

There are three key elements of dancing that stimulate the creativity of the brain. Firstly, dancing raises the heart rate and gets the blood pumping through the arteries; secondly, it changes the way we move; thirdly, it changes our relationship with our physical surroundings. In this chapter I will show how these three elements can activate our cognitive pathways to change the way we think, solve problems and take risks, as well as enhance spatial awareness and mental agility.

Before we start, let's unpack the idea of "creativity." For a word that is used so ubiquitously, it can be hard to quantify. How creative are you? Is creativity measurable? Well, probably not in the truest sense, but there are standard measures, used in psychological testing for employment, and so on, which can at least help to demonstrate how the creative process works. I have included one of these below, a little situation-solution exercise called the Torrance Test of

Creative Thinking, which defines the creative process as comprising four underlying components: fluency, flexibility, originality and elaboration. Have a go!

The situation: Bobby set off for school, but never arrived.

The solution: Give yourself three minutes to write down as many reasons as possible for why Bobby did not arrive at school.

Here are some of the reasons I came up with:

1. Bobby had fallen in love with another student, and they decided to skip school and spend the day in the park.

2. Bobby was run over by a bus.

3. Bobby was run over by a car.

4. Bobby was a dog, who walked to school with his owners every day. Bobby saw a cat, he pulled on his lead, which broke, and he chased the cat around the village pond. His owner was furious. She gave her child to a friend to take to school and spent the next 20 minutes calling Bobby's name. When she got him back on his lead, he was soaking wet, so she took him straight home. That's why Bobby didn't arrive at school.

> 5. Bobby and his dad were driving to school in the snow. They heard on the radio that due to the snow all the schools were closed, so they turned around and went home.

Let's now study the results and work out how creative you are. Start by counting how many reasons you thought of. This is your fluency score. I scored 5 for creative fluency. For your flexibility score, count how many different types of answers you gave. I thought of four different types of answers, as reasons 2 and 3 are essentially the same—he was run over by something. Next, think about how original your answers are, i.e., how unique your answers are compared with the answers you think other people would give. Of my five answers, I would say that three would qualify as original—the idea that Bobby had fallen in love, that he was a dog and that he was driving to school in the snow would probably not be the first thoughts in people's minds, whereas lots of people would likely say that Bobby was run over by something, working on the assumption that people worry about young children and road safety. Finally, to arrive at your creative elaboration score, score each response out of 10 for complexity. My most complex answer is number 4, because I go into a lot of detail about how Bobby is a dog, and there are lots of elements to the story.

LET'S GET CREATIVE

When we move and start to get our hearts pumping, we set off a complex chain of biological events, which can fundamentally change the way we think and solve problems. The first thing that happens is an increase in the rate at which blood is pumped around our body. This is important because a lot of this blood, between 15 and 20% of it, goes to the brain. This is vital, because brain cells will die without the oxygen that the blood carries to them. Blood is like a freight train, transporting things into and out of the brain. In addition to oxygen, it carries carbohydrates, amino acids, fats, hormones and vitamins into the brain and carbon dioxide, ammonia, lactate and hormones away from it.

The dynamic brain is where we do our thinking, and the effective functioning of the brain relies on changes to a variety of molecular, vascular and cellular structures. For example, exercise has been shown to lead to an increase in the production of proteins, such as brain-derived neurotrophic factor, and hormones and neurotransmitters, such as insulin-like growth factor, dopamine and serotonin. Serotonin is known as the happy chemical, because increased production of it can make people feel happier.

The amazing process goes something like this: We move, our hearts pump, our brain gets a shake-up and we feel good. But that's not all. Dancing is different from standard aerobic exercises, such as pedaling away on an exercise bike or running on a treadmill. When we dance, we also stimulate those areas of the brain responsible for a range of mental activities such as spatial awareness, memory, perception, learning and interpersonal cooperation. It is the stimulation of this complex and intricate, interconnected network that underpins the extraordinary link between moving and super-sharp thinking.

Research teams around the world have been studying the links between movement, neurocognitive function and creativity for decades and have made some astonishing findings. What's more, these findings can be applied easily in our everyday lives to make us all a bit more creative.

One study carried out on students at Rhode Island College in the USA found that getting your heart rate pumping is the first step to jump-starting your creative flexibility (i.e., your ability to think of lots of different types of solutions to a given problem).[11] The students had to take a creativity test three times: once after doing nothing physical, once immediately after taking part in 30 minutes of aerobic exercise and once more two hours after the exercise. The researchers found that people were not very creative after doing nothing. However, immediately after 30 minutes of exercise they were super-creative. Amazingly, people were also super-creative when they took the test two hours after doing the exercise, by which time their heart rate had returned to normal.

If you've got to make a decision that involves the need for creative flexibility, such as thinking of a whole new set of imaginative Christmas gifts for your extended family, the best time to draw up a list would be within two hours of getting your heart rate pumping.

In the first chapter, I wrote about how sitting down in a classroom at school felt different from moving freely around the drama and dance studio. I told you how I was never considered smart enough to be put in for exams in geography or history, and that I left school with only one CSE grade 1 in Drama. Interestingly, a study, carried out in London, less than 20 miles from where I went to school, used the contrast between geography and dance as the basis for a scientific study into mood and creativity.

Scientists measured people's mood and creativity immediately after they watched a video about the archeology of the Lake District, and then after they took part in an aerobic dance session.[12] The findings were a perfect replication of my teenage school days: people were in a more positive mood and were more creative following the dance class than following the video session.

If you want to switch off your mind and feel emotionally neutral, then vegging out in front of the TV watching documentaries about rock formation seems to be the perfect thing to do. However, if you would rather feel something more creative and positive, then (to borrow the line from a 1970s kids' TV show) *Why don't you just switch off your television set and go out and do something less boring instead* (like dance)![13]

PROBLEM SOLVING

Not all thinking is the same, just as not all movement is the same. At my research lab, I have found that different types of physical movements affect our ability to think and solve problems in different ways.

There are some problems, for instance, that have just one correct answer, and once you have the answer, that's it: you've arrived at the solution. These are called single-answer problems, and they require "convergent" thinking. Then there are problems with potentially hundreds of correct answers. These multiple-answer problems require "divergent" thinking.

Examples of single-answer questions and convergent thinking

> Q: What's the capital city of France?
> Q: What's 43 × 9?

Just because a question has a single answer doesn't mean that there is a single way of thinking to find the answer. Some single-answer questions require multiple mental steps to work out the solution. Let's think about how you worked out the answer to 43 × 9.

Some people work it out using the following steps:

> Step 1: 43 × 10 = 430
> Step 2: 430 − 43 = 387

Other people use a different set of steps:

> Step 1: 3 × 9 = 27
> Step 2: 40 × 9 = 360
> Step 3: 27 + 360 = 387

Whichever way you do it, you are finding the answer by going through lots of discrete steps. We use this sort of convergent thinking for everyday problem-solving tasks, such as following steps for a recipe or for changing a lightbulb.

Examples of multiple-answer problems and divergent thinking

Q: How would your life be different if you had a long, monkey-like tail?

Q: How many ways are there to change your current exercise routines to give you a healthier lifestyle?

These are problems with lots of right answers rather than just one. Can you think of at least seven alternative uses for a regular household brick? An alternative use is a use for the object for which it was never designed. Some people find this task really hard. People can often only think of three or four alternative uses, but then they tend to get stuck.

This type of problem solving uses divergent thinking because you have to think outside the box; you have to diverge from what is known or expected. Of the hundreds of alternative uses for a brick I have heard, the two that stick in my mind are: to rub a wart off your skin and turned upside down as an ashtray.

I set up an experiment to test the link between

dancing and problem solving in our lab with one of my former graduate students, Carine Lewis.[14] Firstly, we asked our participants to complete a series of divergent and convergent thinking tests. The tests were visual, numerical and language based.

We then split the participants into two groups and asked each to watch and dance along to two different tutorial videos. The first video teaches a structured dance routine. In this video, I am filmed using a range of movements that are simple and coordinated to the regular beat of the music, which the participants are asked to replicate. The second video is an improvised dance session in which I encourage the viewers to focus on one part of their body, for example, their arms, and to copy my improvised arm movements. I then stop moving but ask the participants to carry on with their improvised arm movements until I tell them to move a different body part or move in a different style—like robots, for example, or leaves floating on the wind, or heavy rock music fans.

In the second part of the study, we asked both groups to complete a second set of cognitive and problem-solving tests. When we analyzed the results, we found that the people who had danced to the structured dance video became faster at solving convergent thinking puzzles afterwards. One of the puzzles was a lexical decision task, in which they were given a string of letters, such as "FAMERY," and had to indicate whether they thought the string of letters was a real word or a non-word by pressing one of two buttons on a computer keyboard. They were encouraged to do it as quickly as they could. This task measures how quickly people are able to mentally process visually presented words. What we found was that after 20 minutes of structured dancing, the participants' thought processing sped up, with no loss of accuracy. However, there was no improvement in their divergent or "creative" thinking.

Among the people who did 20 minutes of improvised dancing, there was no increase in their speed of thinking, but we found that they became more creative in the answers they gave to divergent-thinking tasks. For example, before dancing, participants could generate about four or five alternative uses for a common object such as a brick or a newspaper, but after dancing they could generate seven or eight. This is nearly a 100% increase in output.

We are all so caught up in our set patterns of behaving, moving and thinking in our busy lives that it is sometimes difficult to be spontaneous. Don't get me wrong: set patterns of thinking have their uses.

They enable us to predict what we are about to see and hear, they guide us as to how to behave when we go somewhere new and they can help us to resolve ambiguity as we process information from our surroundings. Set patterns of thinking develop with experience; we build them up as we go through life in order to act more efficiently.

Here is an example: imagine you are listening to someone you know speak on a poor telephone line. Even if you can hear only parts of what they are saying, you may be able to piece together the meaning of their words from the context of the conversation and your knowledge of the person who is speaking. In this situation, you are using set patterns of thinking to disambiguate, or fill in missing information.

However, thinking on autopilot has its downsides too. It can result in us getting completely the wrong end of the stick. Stuck in our thinking rut, we find it difficult to be creative and process new information that doesn't fit into a recognizable, set pattern. But change the way you move, and you will change the way you think. Improvised dance shakes up our set patterns of behavior, which in turn helps us to break away from set patterns of thinking. We will look at how to use improvisation in this way later in this chapter.

ME-MOR-IIEEES!

How do dancers remember dance routines? Imagine you have to learn this sequence of dance steps from the page, or better still, have a go at learning it with your body.

Face front.
Start with your feet together.

1. Make a sideways step to the right with your right foot.

2. Make a sideways step to the right with your left foot, crossing your left foot in front of your right.

3. Make a sideways step to the right with your right foot.

4. Tap your left foot on the floor next to your right foot.

5. Make a sideways step to the left with your left foot.

6. Make a sideways step to the left with your right foot, crossing your right foot in front of your left.

7. Make a sideways step to the left with your left foot.

8. Tap your right foot on the floor next to your left foot.

Now repeat this sequence several times.

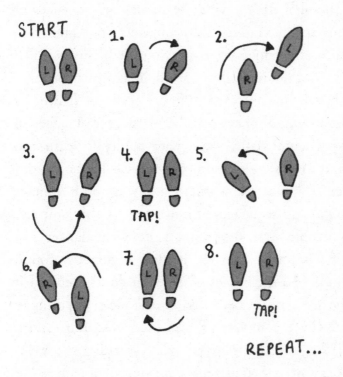

If you have no knowledge of dance, then this small sequence might be hard to learn. However, if you've ever done any line dancing, you will recognize it as a grapevine. It will be encoded in your mind as "doing the grapevine" and as a condensed piece of information it will take up less space and give your memory more opportunity to think about (and learn) other things.

Being familiar with the names of sequences of movements can radically improve your ability to learn and remember dance routines. This is called the "familiarity effect." And it can also be used when trying to learn different styles of dance: by becoming familiar with the physical "language" of a particular dance style, your ability to learn and perform it should improve. Don't be disheartened if you try to learn a new style and you find it difficult to pick up sequences of movements—this is understandable, even if you are a proficient dancer in a different style. Top tip: if there is nobody around to tell you the names of different dance steps, or if the name you've been told doesn't mean anything to you (I was completely flummoxed when I first heard of the "reverse fleckeryl" when learning the Viennese waltz), then just make up your own names; it'll make it much easier to remember them.

Dancers in commercial shows have to learn choreography very quickly. A choreographer will demonstrate the moves, and the dancers will have to learn them simply by watching and repeating what is done, taking correction either from the choreographer or their assistant. During this process, dancers are unlikely to write down what they have to learn; they rely on their visual memory, on what they have learned in the past and what is familiar to them from years of training. As the ballerina Natalia Makarova once put it, "Dancers are trained to 'eat' dances—to ingest them and make them part of who they are. These are physical memories; when dancers know a dance, they know it in their muscles and bones."

First, they have to memorize the movements of the body. These can be broken down into gross motor movements, such as the big gestures involving the limbs, and fine motor movements, those involving the hands and fingers, facial expression, different attitudes within the body and tensions held and released across the body. Dancers also have to remember dozens of other pieces of information, for example, the entrances and exits, the patterns laid out on the floor, their position relative to other dancers. They have to learn how to interact with other people on the stage, so their movements are coordinated in space and time. In addition, they have to learn the music as well as the emotional content of a piece and typically are expected to project all this while taking on the personality of a character. So, as you can see, there are layers of subtlety within the movements, and dancers are expected to learn and remember them all without the aid of a written score.

I love watching *Strictly Come Dancing* on the BBC, and *Dancing with the Stars* when I'm in the USA, as much for the extreme mental processing that the dancers are doing, as for the brilliant performances. And I often think, if only we could see the complex activity going on inside their heads, we would applaud them ten times louder.

To give you an idea of how challenging *Strictly* is, imagine a situation where you had to learn a new language every week, such as Mandarin in Week 1, Russian in Week 2 and Spanish in Week 3 and so on, and you were then tested on your conversational competence in that language in front of eight million people and a panel of linguistic experts. This is what the contestants have to do. Although they are not learning a different spoken language, they are learning a different movement language.

To stick with the linguistic metaphor: it's not just the steps and moves—i.e., the vocabulary and syntax—

that the contestants are having to learn in a very short space of time, but how to speak that language, how to get the body to "pronounce" the words, conjugate the verbs, choose the right idioms to express what they want to say . . .

And it isn't just the celebrity contestants whose brains are working overtime in these dancing shows. The professional dancers sometimes get an extreme mental workout too. In November 2019, Neil Jones, one of the professional dancers, injured his knee just before the live show. What a nightmare—well, it was the Halloween special! But in a scene reminiscent of *42nd Street*, where the star becomes injured and a chorus dancer steps in to save the day and give the performance of her lifetime, another professional, Kevin Clifton, took his place. He learned Neil's dance routine in about 45 minutes and then went out on stage and, with a little help from Alex Scott, his celebrity partner, gave a near-perfect performance. What a star.

Kevin Clifton stepped up to the mark and saved the day. Of course, it was easier for Kevin, as a professional dancer, to learn the whole routine in 45 minutes than it would have been for a less experienced dancer, because Kevin is much more familiar with the language of dance.

If you want to learn dance moves like a pro, there

are two techniques you can use to help improve your memory: marking and sleep.

Marking is a technique used by dancers to help them learn and rehearse sequences of dance movements. It is the opposite of dancing something "full out." Dancing full out means doing everything exactly as it should be done; jumping to full height, turning as many pirouettes as required and fully extending limbs. Marking involves doing the movements in a smaller, energy-conserving way; or replacing one set of movements with another. For example, dancers will often model the exercise with their hands before they do it full out with their feet and legs.

Marking can be a useful technique to conserve energy so that a dancer can get through several hours of rehearsal without becoming physically worn out. There is also evidence that marking can help people learn dance routines because it takes less thinking effort than dancing something full out, so there is some thinking capacity left over for learning and remembering other aspects of the dance.[15]

So what about those other aspects of the dance? Learning some new steps is one thing, but how do you get the body to perform them? How do you control the different parts of the body and move them selectively? You might notice that the judges on shows like *Strictly Come Dancing* often mention how important it is for the dancers to separate the top and bottom halves of their bodies, keeping one part still while the other part is moving. In dance terms, this is called isolation, and in brain terms, it means being able to control activation in one part of the brain while maximizing it in another.

To experience what I'm talking about, next time you walk anywhere, focus on which parts of your body are moving. Then pick a body part, such as an arm, and start walking again, but this time keep that body part perfectly still. How does that feel? Now try it again with another body part and move that part either more slowly or more quickly than normal as you walk. Let's imagine you choose to nod your head: so now you're walking normally with your legs, you're keeping one arm perfectly still and you're nodding your head. How does this feel? You should feel like a dancer. Differentially controlling parts of your body is one of the extraordinary things that dancers learn to do. And it all happens in the motor area of the brain.

The motor area of the brain runs in a strip from the top of your head down towards your ears. Each part controls the movement of a different body part, from your toes to your lips. It's easier to control the movement of some body parts than others because some take up more of the motor area. For example, the movement of our hands and fingers is more important, in terms of motor function, than the movement of our hips and trunk.

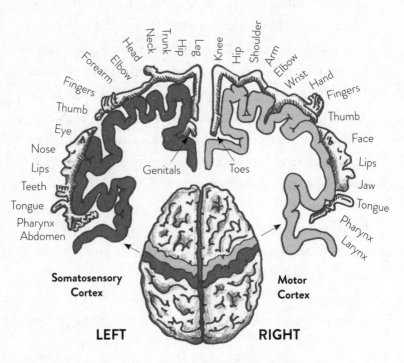

A neurological "map" of the areas of the human brain dedicated to processing motor functions, or sensory functions, for different parts of the body. Note that the size of each region is related not to its actual size, but to the complexity of the movements it can perform.

As dancers, we need to overcome the inherent limitations of the motor area and have equal levels of control over all body parts. If you're a lindy hopper, learn some kathak, or if you're a devoted bun-head, experience what it feels like to learn a bit of hoedown.

And, ideally, do it not in the morning, or in the evening, but at bedtime! Which brings us to the other technique for improving the memory. Scientists agree that the best time to learn a dance routine, or indeed anything, is before you go to sleep.

This is because the brain builds new knowledge structures, called "schemas," while we sleep, and it is these structures that underpin our ability to learn and remember information.

In 2002, a team of scientists from the Laboratory of Neuroscience at Harvard Medical School were particularly interested in this idea and decided to explore the effect of sleeping on people's memory for movements.[16] They taught people a finger-dance—a sequence of movements with just one finger—and then assessed how well they could remember it twelve hours later. The results were amazing. The people who learned the dance and then slept before being tested performed it much better than those who learned it and then stayed awake before being tested. What is even more remarkable is that it doesn't matter when you sleep—you still get the same improvement in performance even if you learn something, then wait all day before going to bed. The important point is that the improvement in performance comes after you have slept. If ever you find yourself in a situation where you have to learn a sequence of body movements, be patient with yourself, and sleep. When you wake up, your brain will have consolidated the movements, and your performance will be better.

It is thought that consolidation in memory is facilitated by communication between different regions of the brain, in particular the hippocampus and the neocortex. The hippocampus houses the short-term memory system; it is a place where we process new information, or information we are currently thinking about. New information needs to be integrated into our long-term memory structures in order for us to retain it. This takes place within the neocortex, the outer layer of the brain. Although information fades away from short-term or working memory quite quickly, consolidation into long-term memory can preserve information for a lifetime.

I can still remember dance routines that I learned in my teens, and this is because all the information about those dance routines has been consolidated into my long-term knowledge structures.

PARKINSON'S

One of the most astounding scientific findings about dance came to my attention in 2007, when a group of physiotherapists reported the results of a study based on tango dancing and the neurological condition Parkinson's.[17] They found that when people with Parkinson's took part in a series of partnered tango dance classes, their physical symptoms improved remarkably. People with Parkinson's don't have enough of a chemical called dopamine, because the cells that produce it have stopped working properly, giving rise to a series of both physical and mental symptoms, such as loss of balance, tremors, stiffness and slowness of movement, impaired thinking, pain, anxiety and depression.

When I heard about this finding, I was skeptical. I simply didn't believe that symptoms caused by neurodegeneration could be improved by a few sessions of tango dancing. However, because I have seen the amazing power of dance to help people who suffer from a multitude of different conditions, I was intrigued enough to test the finding myself. I put together a team of top scientists, including a neuroscientist, a physiotherapist, a cognitive psychologist, an occupational therapist and a social anthropologist, and experts in improvised dance, ballet, ballroom and show dance, and set up a lab to investigate.[18]

The original research in this area had shown that dancing could help with the *physical* symptoms of Parkinson's, such as balance and walking, and I wanted to see if others would be alleviated too. I wanted to look at the effects of dancing on thinking and problem solving, quality of life and depression.

On the first day of the study, we assessed a group of men and women with Parkinson's on a wide range of physical abilities, as well as thinking and problem-solving skills and quality of life. A few days later, our volunteers started to dance. They took part in twice-weekly sessions of contact improvisation. At the end of the first session, most complained that this wasn't dance. Rolling around on the floor, leaning against the wall and intertwining and moving their arms around with another person, to the sound of whales mating, wasn't what they were expecting. We were worried that none of them would come back for the second session, but they did. In the name of science, they all came back for more, and by the end of ten sessions they were all loving the freedom of contact improvisation. A few days after their final dance session, we assessed everyone again on the same measures as before, and what we found was extraordinary.

One of the tests we performed involved timing how long it took people to stand up from a chair and walk a certain distance. These movements are often impaired in people with Parkinson's as the neuro-degeneration slows them down and affects their balance. We found that after ten sessions of contact improvisation, the participants were much faster at this fundamentally important physical task. Another of our tests looked at people's emotional well-being and bodily discomfort, and both had improved considerably over the course of the study. Finally, we were amazed to see improvements in the way people thought about and solved problems. The dancing, or rolling on the floor to whale sounds, had made them think differently and more creatively.

Everyone in the research team was stunned, but as skeptical scientists, we knew we shouldn't get too carried away too soon. We sat around a table and decided that we should run all the tests again, just to be sure. So we set up another study, recruited more people with Parkinson's and changed the style of dance. This time we led people through characterful dances, such as the Charleston, a Bollywood routine, a Cockney knees-up and some Saturday Night Fever, all to music that had a very strong rhythmic beat. We also measured everyone's mood at several points before, during and after the sessions. After twelve weeks, we were delighted to find the same improvements in people's physical functions and quality of life, and what's more, for the first time, we found a reduction in feelings of depression, anger and tension and an increase in vigor. People felt happier and less tired after an hour of bopping along to a beat.

So the message is: whatever state you are in, do your body and mind a favor and dance. The movements don't have to be complex or challenging. Take the wonderful story of Helen Keller's visit with the famous dancer Martha Graham. Keller, an American author and activist who was both deaf and blind, met Graham in her dance studio. Feeling the vibrations of the dancers' movements on the floor, Keller asked what they were doing. "Jumping," said Graham. To which Keller replied, "What is jumping?" Graham then asked one of her dancers, Merce Cunningham, to stand at the barre and gently placed Keller's hands on his waist. As he jumped, Keller followed the movements with her fingers, feeling his muscles flexing and releasing, experiencing all the motions of his body as he moved up and down. In her autobiography, Graham recalls that Keller's "expression changed from curiosity to one of joy. You could see the enthusiasm rise in her face as she threw her arms in the air." When

Merce stopped, Keller exclaimed, "Oh, how wonderful! How like thought! How like the mind it is."

Dancing, like thinking, allows us to flex muscles that transcend a purely physical realm—it affects our social, cognitive and emotional health, which means that, when we dance, we give a boost to all these aspects of our lives.

THE POWER OF IMPROVISATION

Let's look at what happens when, rather than following a familiar routine or repeating a dance we know well, we force ourselves to let go, dance freestyle, with no agenda or structure. How does this impact our brain and the way we think?

Improvisation is the act of creating something new, extemporaneously—that is, without planning or preparation. Engaging in improvisation has a fundamental effect on the way people think in all walks of life. When we improvise, our brain does a full-blown mental workout; we need to access a broad base of knowledge and be creative, innovative and flexible. This can be difficult because we are so used to planning everything we do, or acting in a way prescribed by someone else. Improvisation requires that our actions are guided by intuition, where intuition is the rapid processing of experienced information. It doesn't have to be complicated. To try it right now, just put on some music and move a part of your body in a way you've never moved it before.

Improvisation techniques are used frequently in music, drama, dance and other arts, and there is an increasing trend to apply them in other areas, such as business, education and training, product development and health. When comparing experts with novices, one of the biggest differentiators is the ability to improvise. For example, Carol Livingston and Hilda Borko, two US educators, claim that the ability to improvise is a feature that differentiates expert teachers from novice teachers.[19] They report that expert teachers use improvisation techniques while teaching to a greater extent than novice teachers because they are able to make use of extensive networks of easily accessible information, which enables them to quickly select strategies, explanations, routines and relevant information in real time while the lesson progresses in a dynamic way. Improvisation frees the expert teacher from having to stick to a script and allows them to meet the needs of students more flexibly as and when they arise. Improvisational skills are vital in business too, enabling people to identify and exploit opportunities to create novel products and ways of doing business. Having worked with many businesses, I have seen how those with the confidence and know-how to improvise achieve amazing results.

Dancing is a great way to practice improvisation because you don't need any special skills or equipment. All you have to do is try something with your body that you have never done before. For example, try walking with an extra wiggle of the hips, or a strut, or make new patterns with your arms by waving them in the air in a unique way. Sometimes it's easier to improvise by taking inspiration from the movements you see in nature, or from a piece of music. Or, if you're feeling really adventurous, you could take inspiration from the American choreographer and artist Remy Charlip, who once spoke on a radio show about a do-it-yourself dance instructional manual he dreamed of making:

It would be called *Dances Any Body Can Do*. And they would be mostly household dances, like, dance in a doorway, dance on the stairs, dance in a bed, and other dances that you can do that would be very simple. And I'd like to do a second book . . . called *More Advanced Dances*, which would be very difficult to do, like dancing on the tip of a candle flame, or dancing on a cloud . . .

Why not give it a go? You'll be amazed at the results!

STANDING STILL

In 1990, Madonna released a song called "Vogue," whose opening line is "Strike a pose." The basic premise of the song is that if you want to escape the pain of life and be something else, something better, then you should lose yourself on the dance floor, the idea being that "striking a pose" can help you unlock your imagination, where you'll find inner beauty and inspiration. Of course, this is just a pop song, but several scientific studies seem to show that striking a pose (or standing in a particular way) can change the way people think and feel.

One of the most influential psychological studies published so far this century was carried out by Dana Carney, Amy Cuddy and Andy Yap at Columbia and Harvard Universities in 2010.[20] Forty-two people were divided into two groups and made to stand or sit in a number of poses. The people in the first group were placed in "high-power poses." A high-power pose is a way of standing or sitting that looks confident, relaxed and self-assured. Imagine leaning back in your chair, with your arms behind your head and your feet up on the desk in front of you, or leaning over a desk with your arms spread wide. The people in the second group were placed in "low-power poses," which are poses that look closed and constricted. Imagine sitting on a chair with both feet flat on the floor and your hands crossed over your lap or standing with your legs and arms crossed. All the participants were asked to hold their poses for a total of two minutes.

The research team took three measurements. First, they asked the participants how "powerful" and "in charge" they felt. Perhaps unsurprisingly, those who had been standing or sitting in high-power poses felt more powerful and more in charge than those who'd been standing or sitting in low-power poses.

Secondly, they set the participants a "risk-taking" gambling task. People were given $2 and a dice. They could either keep the money (the safe bet) or they could roll the dice (the high-risk bet). If they rolled the dice and got an odd number, they lost the $2. However, if they rolled an even number, they won $4. What would you do? The scientists found that 86% of those people who had been placed in the high-power poses took the high-risk bet, compared to only 60% of the people placed in the low-power poses. It seems to be the case that just standing or sitting in a particular pose for a couple of minutes is enough to change how powerful people feel and also influences their risk-taking behavior. This implies that if you want to take a risk and you need to get into a riskier mindset, you should strike a powerful pose first.

What I find really amazing is the researchers' third finding. Before the participants took up their poses, each had to provide a saliva sample, which was used to measure concentrations of the stress hormone cortisol and the sex hormone testosterone in their bodies. It is thought that these hormones are markers of dominance/leadership in a person, testosterone indicating a high level and cortisol a low level. Once the participants had finished posing, they provided a second saliva sample. The researchers found that in the people in the high-power posing group, testosterone levels had gone up and cortisol levels had gone down, whereas in the people in the low-power posing group, testosterone levels had gone down and cortisol levels had gone up. So stationary postures not only affect how we think about ourselves but also influence our hormonal state. Standing or sitting in a particular way for just two minutes has a profound effect on us. I always knew this as a teenager; sitting hunched over a desk at school made me feel powerless and stressed, whereas standing in the drama studio with my shoulders back made me feel in control, relaxed and prepared to take risks and try something new.

LEAP BEFORE YOU LOOK

Just as improvised dancing pushes the brain out of its comfort zone to think spontaneously, so changing the space and environment we move in can inspire us to think in new ways.

To prove this, I have devised a simple experiment you can try at home. Below are two problems to solve. Read them, follow my movement instructions and then try to solve the problems.

Problem 1: Nine dots

Here are nine dots. Can you draw four straight lines to connect all the dots, keeping your pen on the page?

O   O   O

O   O   O

O   O   O

Problem 2: Brothers

Imagine you're walking home late one night and feel lost. You get to a T-intersection and are unsure which direction to take. At the junction are two people, brothers John and David. You know two things about them: one, they both know which way you have to go to get home; and two, one of them always tells the truth, and the other always lies, but you don't know which is which. You have one chance to ask them just one question. What single question do you ask to guarantee that you get the information you need to find your way home?

Now before trying to work these problems out, I want you to stand up and walk around the room in a random pattern for a few minutes. Don't walk in straight lines around the edge of the room; instead, change your direction every few steps—turn right, then left, make big looping turns and small, sharp turns. Now, see if you can work out the answers.

Solutions

Most people fail to find a solution to the nine-dot problem because they think "inside the box." They try to find ways of connecting the nine dots by drawing only within the space of the nine dots, as if the dots on the outer edge of the "square" form a boundary that mustn't be crossed. To solve this problem, you must think "outside the box," literally, because you have to draw lines which go beyond what you perceive to be the boundary of the problem.

Here's the solution:

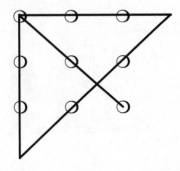

To solve the brothers problem, you have to come at it from a counterintuitive position. You want the truth, but you don't know who will tell you the truth. Therefore, there is no point asking either of the brothers for the truthful answer to your question, because you won't know for certain if it's true or false. You must ask a question that you know will give you the incorrect answer and then do the opposite of what they say. Let's assume that John always tells the truth and David always lies. You can only ask one question, so addressing either one of the brothers, the best question to ask is: Which way would your brother say is the correct way home? You need to factor in the lie and then do the opposite.

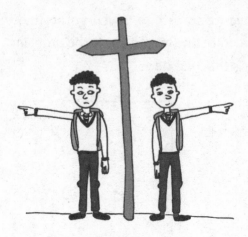

A group of scientists from Singapore, New York and Michigan published a study in 2012 that backs up the experiment you have just performed.[21] They asked people to either walk around the perimeter of a square for two minutes or walk freely, in any way they liked, around a room. Remarkably, they found that the subjects' thinking was affected by the way they walked. Those who walked freely around the room scored higher in tests to measure creative originality than those who were constrained and could only walk around the perimeter.

Next time you walk to the store or move around your office or school, try to find a new route, or walk in a different pattern, and then see what new things you notice. Look up, or down, walk backwards, sideways, zigzag and change direction. Walk upstairs as if you're on the set of a 1950s MGM musical, or you're Rocky Balboa in training for a big fight. Then make a list of all the things you've walked past hundreds of times before and never noticed. It doesn't matter how big or small the things are; just note them and realize how much of the world we don't see, even though it's right under our noses.

You will find that varying your environment and how you move through it can work wonders on your brain. Your creative mind will switch on, and you will start to see the world differently and think more imaginatively.

RUGBY AND THE PAS DE BOURRÉE

A few years ago, I undertook an experiment that nicely demonstrated the cognitive and creative benefits of dance. This experiment, commissioned by Channel 4, was part of a pilot for a new TV show called *Dr. Dance*. The aim was to see if I could improve people's performance in a range of tasks by teaching them different forms of dance, and I was challenged to take a failing and dispirited semi-professional rugby league team and see if I could turn them into a winning side.

The director and I arrived in Greater Manchester on a Sunday afternoon to watch our team lose. At first glance, they were slow, heavy-footed, and seemed not to know each other's names or how to function efficiently as a team. After watching them play and train, I knew that I could help to improve their performance by addressing three aspects of their game: teamwork, spatial awareness and agility, all of which are fundamental to dancing too.

Being semi-professional meant that they all had full-time jobs outside of playing rugby and could only train on weeknights and play matches on the weekend. To help the team bond as a group, I set up weekly dance classes. As I discussed earlier, moving together on a shared rhythm can lead to increased levels of pro-social (i.e., helpful) behaviors and enhance social bonding. The team was so busy training that they neglected one of the most important aspects of playing a team sport: working together and developing as a social unit.

I introduced the team to folk and country dances to demonstrate the principles of group spatial awareness and orientation. I chose these dances because they were similar in structure to what players do on the rugby pitch and had similar demands. On the pitch, the rugby players have to move forward in lines, keeping a loose and flexible formation; they have to dodge around their opponents and they have to maintain synchronicity and timing so they can pass the ball between themselves and keep it from members of the other team. In the folk and country dances I chose, a line of men, holding hands, skipped towards and away from a line of women and then walked through arches made by the women, and turned around, before holding hands with each other again to make arches for the women to walk through. The dances were carried out to music.

Most of the team engaged with the exercise. It was a fun and practical way for them to experience the mechanics of good teamwork, without having to get muddy on the rugby pitch. There was, however, one player who sat obstinately on the sidelines and refused to take part. The player with the fear of dancing was the winger. Built like a 1970s Volvo station wagon, solid with the turning circle of a super-tanker, he could knock anyone over, but he wasn't quick enough to dodge around them. When I asked why he didn't want to join in, he told me that he thought skipping was beneath his professional level. This is fair enough: some people just don't want to dance, and I would never try to force anyone to do something that made them feel uncomfortable. However, the winger's reluctance to join in with the skipping seemed at odds with what I'd noticed during his on-pitch training a few days earlier, when he'd thrown himself wholeheartedly into a warm-up exercise that looked remarkably like skipping.

On the days following the folk-dance session, I chatted with the winger about his aim to become a more agile rugby player. I pointed out the similarities between his on-pitch warm-up exercises and the movements involved in dancing. I wanted him to see firsthand the parallels between professional male ballet dancers and professional male rugby players; both are fast, incredibly strong and, most of all, exceptionally agile. So I arranged for the winger to attend an advanced-level male ballet class at the Northern Ballet School in Manchester, one of the top ballet schools in the country, to try out their techniques to enhance agility. The ballet dancers had very different physical frames compared to the chunky winger. They too were muscular and strong, but they were also lean and flexible, more racehorse than draft horse; the perfect physique for optimum agility. Therefore, it was no surprise that in a series of jumping exercises, the ballet dancers leaped and darted with power and urgency while the winger struggled. It was in these areas—power, urgency and, most of all, agility—that the winger needed to improve.

The lightbulb moment for the winger came when the ballet master demonstrated a fast series of steps known as a *pas de bourrée*, a sideways step in which one foot passes either in front or behind the other. The winger recognized this as a more intricate and faster version of a training exercise his squad practiced with a rope ladder. Wearing ballet shoes, he was able to feel the whole movement in different parts of his feet, particularly through the balls of his feet. He felt more in control of his body. This was due to an enhanced level of proprioceptive feedback from his feet. Proprioception is the body's ability to sense movement from sensory receptors in muscles, joints, tendons and skin. Proprioceptive feedback signals are sent to the brain, providing information on the current position of different body parts and how they move and change location over time.

To give yourself a sense of how this works, try the following simple exercise:

- Stretch one arm out to the side.

- Stretch the other arm high above your head.

- Point the index finger of both hands.

- Close your eyes and then, keeping your eyes closed, move both hands in front of you and touch the tips of your index fingers together.

You are able to do this action because proprioceptive feedback signals are being sent by your moving limbs so that your brain knows exactly where each index finger is in space and time and can therefore navigate them together, even when your eyes are closed.

An increase in proprioceptive feedback, particularly through the feet, increases your agility because you have more information about where your feet are and what they are doing, which will give you greater control of your movements. That's why it's sometimes important to take off a pair of heavy boots or shoes and feel the floor beneath your feet.

Following the winger's enlightenment, we took the *pas de bourrée* exercise back to the rugby training ground and made two simple changes to the team's ladder training exercise: they took off their rugby boots for a small part of the exercise to experience feeling the earth beneath their feet, and they varied the speed and rhythm at which they performed it.

Focusing on these three simple adjustments to an established training regime—teamwork, spatial awareness and agility—the players started to play as a team and win. Their spatial awareness improved, which gave them a group dynamic and helped them to function as a well-oiled machine. The winger found a new way to dodge and side-step other players, which was much more effective than trying to run through solid bodies. The team's performance and position in the league slowly improved, and as the season went on, they were promoted to the league above. The winger is now happy to skip.

Who knew that burly rugby players and sinewy, supple dancers had so much in common? Certainly, watching rugby can be very like watching dance. They both consist of beautiful movements with patterns and sequences. In rugby, there are even points where one player is lifted high into the air. The whole experiment was a thoroughly rewarding and enlightening experience for me. And the more I understood the dynamics of the game, the more I grew to appreciate the shapes of its movement on the pitch.

As the philosopher Alan W. Watts put it: "The

only way to make sense out of change is to plunge into it, move with it, and join the dance." This philosophy speaks to my own experience of how dance can be a catalyst for changing human behavior. My number one take-home message is simply this: if you want to make changes to the way you think, then start with the way you move your body.

CHAPTER 4

EMOTIONS IN MOTION

"I dance to release endorphins and make me happy.
I dance to share joy and laugh with others.
I dance to feel my heart beat faster."
—Female, aged 23, Dr. Dance Survey:
"Why Do You Dance?"

I have often been so overwhelmed with emotion when dancing that I have cried. There is a jazz class I attend at Pineapple dance studios, which starts with a stretch, deep breaths and loud music. We breathe in and stretch up, before we release from the stretch and exhale. It is on the changeover from inhale to exhale that the emotion catches me, and I have to swallow hard to suppress the free flow of tears. It's a moment that marks the beginning of an hour-long catharsis, a period of emotional purging. The warm-up and stretch last for about 30 minutes and then Fleur, the instructor, teaches a routine that is full of expression.

The body is brilliant at communicating emotion, but other than in a dance class, where do we get the chance to act out with our body what is going on deep in our heart? Most of our lives are spent disconnecting our emotions from our physical expression of them. We feel things, but we cannot express them. Unless you're a 6-year-old child, or a Labrador, you cannot freely and spontaneously physically express yourself. Dancing gives humans a tail to wag. In Fleur's jazz class I have a tail, and I wag it.

We learn routines of different styles, some slow and lyrical, others fast and outward-looking. The two styles speak to different emotional connections between the body and the rest of the world. The lyrical routines seem to amplify the intensity of our emotional states: love, loss, disappointment, hope, determination, strength, ambition, pride, jealousy, resilience. These emotions are drawn out as we sweat and are left, literally, on the dance studio floor. We collapse to the floor, roll and grow upwards, peeling ourselves away from everything that is holding us back. We feel the emotion of the dance deep inside, and although we are in a large studio full of other people, there is a feeling of personal isolation. We are dancing for ourselves; we have connected with our innermost feelings, which spill out into the body in movements that are almost subconscious. It is no wonder that people feel emotional when they dance.

During fast routines there is a completely different focus. Then it is as if we have a superpower that enables us to produce fireballs of passion to tell the world exactly who we are and how we are feeling. Sometimes the routines are a combination of both fast and lyrical, and then the class whips itself up into an expressive and cathartic climax.

This emotional high we get from dancing is down to dopamine, the brain chemical I talked about in the section about Parkinson's in the last chapter. As we saw, as well as having an effect on movement, dopamine plays a role in how we feel, and low levels of dopamine are associated with feelings of anxiety, hopelessness, fatigue, demotivation, pain, lack of energy and mood swings. Dancing to music is a great way to overcome these negative feelings because both the exercise and our emotional responses to the music we're hearing can increase the release of dopamine in different parts of the brain. As dopamine levels go up, we can shake off some of those negative feelings and float into a euphoric state.

The lowest periods in my life have been when I've stopped dancing. I was a fool when I stopped to study for my higher degrees. Had I known then what I know now about moving and thinking, I would have danced every day. I remember attending an Argentine tango session after a long break from dance and finding it complicated and difficult but intoxicating. I went to bed on a high and woke up smiling with aching cheeks. Over the years I've learned to self-medicate with dance to keep my mood stable.

DANCE YOUR BLUES AWAY

Depression can be overwhelming and all-consuming. When you are in the throes of it, it can become increasingly difficult to switch off negative thoughts, leaving insufficient headspace to think about other things. Dancing helps to switch off these thoughts and encourages people to concentrate, learn and remember new things.

And there is plenty of science to back this up. One study, carried out in Germany, examined the effects of dance on people who had been admitted to a psychiatric hospital with depression.[22] It was found that just one 30-minute session of dance was enough to reduce their symptoms and increase feelings of vitality. The study used a lively, upbeat dance called the Hava Nagila, which means "let us rejoice" in Hebrew. It involves some quite lively, energetic dancing in a circle to uplifting music. After completing the study, the researchers wanted to know whether it was the music on its own that was causing the reduction in depressive symptoms, so they conducted another trial in which a second group of people with depression just sat and listened to the music. In this music-only group, the patients actually became slightly more depressed! So it seems that dancing is key. And it's remarkable that just one 30-minute session is sufficient to lead to observable results.

In another study, this time carried out in Korea, scientists wanted to know whether a longer-term program of dance would lead to improvements in mood in a group of 16-year-old schoolgirls who had mild depression.[23] The girls were divided into two groups. One group took part in three dance sessions a week for twelve weeks, and the other group, the control group, did nothing. The dance sessions were focused on body awareness, movement and expressing feelings and images. The scientists found that, as might be expected, there was no change in mood for the girls in the control group, whereas the dancing sessions led to a reduction in feelings of depression, anxiety and hostility for the other group. The scientists attributed this improvement in symptoms to the fact that dance made the girls feel more physically relaxed, thus diluting the concentration of stress hormones circulating around their bodies.

What is interesting about both these studies is that different types of dancing, lively and energetic in the first study, reflective and expressive in the second, have a positive impact on the mood of people with both severe and mild depression. And it seems that the more depressed you are, the greater the impact dancing will have.

Two researchers from the UK, Andrew Lane and David Lovejoy, gave 80 people a questionnaire that assessed emotions such as tension, anger, fatigue, depression, vigor and confusion, and grouped the participants according to how depressed they were.[24] Participants were grouped into either a "no-depression group" or a "depressed mood group" using pre-exercise depression scores. Then everyone took part in a 60-minute aerobic dance session. After the dance session, they completed the questionnaire again. The results showed that, following the dance class, there was a general reduction across the board in feelings of anger, confusion, fatigue and tension, but the reduction was greater in the depressed mood group.

One of the greatest success stories I've heard about the positive changes in mood and emotions brought about by dance comes from a program in Edinburgh. A group of dance teachers invited recovering addicts to an early-evening Zumba class. Adults who have been addicted to substances such as drugs and alcohol often say they miss the sensation of being high and feel emotionally flat. The Zumba class allowed the (mostly male) attendees to experience an intense and entirely natural high. It was transformational for their mood. Arriving low and pent up, they would leave open and invigorated.

SELF-ESTEEM AND CONFIDENCE

The poet Kamand Kojouri writes that we dance "to fall in love with ourselves," and this is something that I've observed throughout my dancing and teaching career. Time and again, dancers have told me how much of an impact dancing has had on their sense of self-worth.

A report published by the Health Development Agency in 2000 following research into the link between participation in the arts and health found that engaging in arts-based activities definitely improved participants' sense of well-being and self-esteem.[25] Across 90 projects, 91% reported a development in people's self-esteem, and 82% reported increased confidence.

Wouldn't it be wonderful if we could set up more places where communities could come together through dance, in airports, parks, on high streets and in doctors' offices? We are, supposedly, in the middle of an anxiety epidemic in the UK, in which people are suffocating under the weight of low self-esteem and lack of confidence. Wouldn't it be great if we could reduce this burden through more community dance?

A research study carried out in Manchester, which looked at the impact of dance and swimming on body image satisfaction and physical self-perceptions, recruited a group of girls between the ages of 13 and 14 who were all dissatisfied with their body image, and who didn't do very much exercise.[26] The girls were divided into two groups—a dancing group and a swimming group—and asked to carry out their designated activity twice a week for six weeks. At the end of the study, the girls in the dancing group reported huge positive changes in their perception of their physical worth and attractiveness, and also dramatic reductions in their sense of feeling fat. For the girls in the swimming group, however, there were no changes in any of these areas. These girls continued to feel just as dissatisfied with their body image as they had six weeks earlier.

This is why I am such a strong advocate of dance for emotional well-being. More than any other form of exercise, it has the power to transform how we feel about ourselves.

POWER AND FEELING EMPOWERED

There are times when dance is used explicitly and purposefully as a means of expressing aggression and intimidation. Let's consider a dance that has mesmerized crowds at rugby stadiums around the world, including Twickenham, the home of British rugby. The dance is the haka, and the New Zealand All Blacks perform it before every international match.

The dance involves facial contortions, sticking out your tongue, making your eyes bulge, stamping your feet and slapping your body, and can be accompanied by cries, grunts and chanted words. The haka gives the rugby team energy, and it makes the players feel powerful. It also instills fear in the opposition, just as it would have done when it was danced before battles to the death.

The haka is historically a war dance: an ancient posture dance performed by the Maori, the indigenous people of New Zealand, before going into battle. There are several varieties, including the "peruperu," a choreographed dance to evoke the god of war and to give opponents one last chance to back out, and the "neri," an un-choreographed dance performed to motivate people psychologically. One of the purposes of the haka was to unify the dancers, to put them in a single frame of mind. War dances that were well organized and executed in perfect time by all the dancers (warriors) were considered lucky. It is thought that the dances were passed down from one generation to the next—they may have originated as early as the thirteenth century, when the first Polynesian settlers arrived in New Zealand.

For the All Blacks, the aim of the haka is to intimidate their opponents and make themselves feel united as a team, powerful and invincible. Some of the movements, such as the throat-slitting gestures, had to be removed in 2006 because they were considered just a bit too aggressive. While the All Blacks are probably the most famous pre-match-dancing rugby team, they are certainly not the only ones to perform the haka: rugby teams from Fiji, Samoa and Tonga use a similar tactic to empower themselves.

Scientists in Japan and New Zealand have examined the impact dancing the haka has on people's psychological and emotional state.[27] After the performance, haka dancers report feeling excited and provocative, and experiencing a sense of motivational dominance. People have known for centuries that moving your body in a particular way can successfully prepare you for battle. The way opposing rugby teams deal with the haka varies considerably. Some just stand and watch in fear, some avert their eyes, while others defiantly stare them down at very close quarters.

Never underestimate the power of the human body to communicate emotions and generate a response in others: we stimulate the brains of those watching us when we move in different ways, and as we change the emotions that underpin our movements, we activate different areas of our observers' brains. Imagine you're watching an emotional movie, one in which the actors convey happiness, followed by fear, then sadness: you'll be getting a full-on brain workout as you process all this information. My emotional movie for this full-on brain workout is *Singin' in the Rain*.

COMMUNICATING EMOTION— AN ARTIST'S APPROACH

I've always been entranced when choreographers and dancers succeed in changing the way I feel. The first time I remember this happening was at a ballet performance of *Romeo and Juliet* (choreographed by Kenneth MacMillan). I was touched by the tenderness and love of Juliet and Romeo as they kissed on the bed. It was almost as if the couple weren't dancing, and I felt awkward, like a voyeur, spying on their intimacy. It was a beautiful portrayal, and it moved me.

Romeo and Juliet was the inspiration for the musical *West Side Story*, and the dancing in this film also made a big impact on me emotionally. The choreography, by Jerome Robbins, embodies and communicates perfectly the different emotional states of the Jets and the Sharks. In one routine, danced to Stephen Sondheim's "Cool," we can feel the pent-up frustration in the tight, sharp, staccato movements, as Riff's anger is expressed in an explosive physical release of muscles and limbs, and echoed in the movements of the rest of his gang.

This is a great example of how a solely scientific explanation can fall short of capturing the essence of real emotional expression and communication. Partly, this is because it is extremely rare that we ever feel just one single emotion. For example, when people are feeling happy, they may also experience simultaneous feelings of guilt, or when they are feeling proud they may also have a sense of embarrassment. Our emotions run through us like rivers. And it is for this reason that scientists won't always find the answer to deeply psychological questions about dancing and/or emotions by academic investigation. Great art and the human experience cannot always be dissected by science. Scientists generally rely on words to document, describe and disseminate their observations, and because emotions and art are more powerful than words, they often transcend what scientists can glean from their experiments.

CHAPTER 5

WHAT STOPS PEOPLE FROM DANCING

"We are more often frightened than hurt;
and we suffer more from imagination
than from reality."

—Lucius Annaeus Seneca

Dancing, as we have seen, is so good for physical and mental well-being because it has lots of elements that, when combined, can address the needs of all age groups, both to maintain good health and to assist in the recovery from illness. It can be fun, expressive, challenging, stimulating and sociable.

There are, however, a number of things that stand in the way of people getting all the health and well-being benefits of dancing. These include lack of confidence, lack of motivation, fear of the amount of effort involved and whether they will be up to it. Well, let me tell you, if any of these things are getting in the way of you dancing, read on, because I'm going to show you that you can dance regardless of your physical abilities and help you understand that dancing is for everyone. Yes, everyone.

DANCING AND SELF-ESTEEM

Some years ago, I carried out a study—a Dr. Dance survey—of around 14,000 people, exploring people's level of dance confidence and the impact of age and sex on the way dance confidence changes across our lifespan.[28] Here's the scene I set and what I asked:

Imagine you're at a party, nightclub or wedding where you're dancing along with other people. Imagine you're dancing to your favorite piece of music. You're in your groove and feeling great. As you look around the room, you notice that everyone else who's dancing is the same age and sex as you. How are they dancing? Now, answer the following question. Compared to other people of your own age and gender, how good a dancer do you think you are? I don't mean how accomplished you are in terms of technique or achievements in a particular style of dance (such as ballroom or lindy hop); I mean how confident do you feel about just letting yourself go and moving to the music? Give yourself a score between 1 and 7, where 1 is terrible and 7 is fantastic.

Your response to this question will be influenced by two ways of thinking. Firstly, by how competent, or how good, you think you are at dancing, and secondly, by how you think other people view your dancing (this is called "reflected appraisal").

Many factors will have come into play in your assessment. However, the two that will have had the greatest effect are your age and sex.

Self-esteem has been found to change at key developmental periods of our lives. So, for both men and women, general self-esteem is higher in younger teenagers, below the age of 18, than in the early adulthood group between the ages of 18 and 22. At this point, self-esteem stabilizes and then appears not to change between the ages 23 and 49. It then rises steadily during our fifties and sixties before it drops again in our seventies and eighties.

Although age affects self-esteem in both sexes in a similar way, there are well-established differences between men and women that influence their dance confidence. In general, men tend to have higher self-esteem than women. Although women tend to have higher self-esteem than men regarding their behavioral conduct, morals and ethics, they have lower self-esteem than men regarding their physical appearance, athleticism, and personal self-satisfaction.

In my study I found dance-confidence self-esteem changes as people get older and that generally it is higher in women than in men, but there were some surprises. Here's what I found.

Although levels of dance-confidence self-esteem were very high in girls below the age of 16, they dropped dramatically in early adulthood, to almost the lowest point in a woman's life. But why should this be the case? One possible reason is competency. Let's assume that girls and young adult women use recreational dance for different purposes, and this change in purpose reflects a change in their competence at social dance. For girls under 16, recreational dance is simply a fun, enjoyable activity. They might either dance on their own at home or in small groups with other girls, or they might attend formal dance classes. All these activities increase their dance confidence because young girls are accomplished and competent at using dance for these purposes. Around the age of 16, girls often give up formal dance classes. I have asked hundreds of girls about their dance history, and of those who had stopped dancing, most had stopped taking formal dance classes between the ages of 15 and 18. At about the same time, young women are likely to start dancing publicly in front of members of the opposite sex at parties. When young women start dancing in this way, publicly, they are not accomplished in this use of social recreational dance, especially when they first embark on it, which might explain why they have lower levels of dance confidence.

Competency may also account for the low levels of dance confidence I have seen in boys under the age of 16 and in the steady increase in dance-confidence self-esteem that I have seen as boys get older. Boys under the age of 16 do not enjoy the same advantage of high dance-confidence self-esteem as girls of the same age because they do not, on the whole, use dance in the same way as girls during this period of their development. Young boys are less likely to dance with male friends at home, and they are less likely to enroll in formal dance classes than girls.

However, there tends to be a rise in dance confidence in young men in their late teens and early twenties. According to Charles Darwin, one function of social dance for young men is as a courtship display. Social recreational dance is therefore part of the sexual-selection, or mate-selection, process. According to this view, young men dance for two reasons: to display themselves to potential mates and to make themselves stand out from their mate-selection competitors. The way young men dance, and the way they are perceived by women, is related to both their hormonal make-up and their genetic quality. In social-dance settings, such as discos and nightclubs, men are clearly being watched and evaluated as potential mates. This evaluation is just the type of social feedback that will have an impact on a person's dance-confidence self-esteem. As men and women use dance more and more as part of the mate-selection process during their late teens and early twenties, both sexes will become more competent with this function of dance and both will get used to receiving feedback from other people, which leads to higher ratings of dance confidence. We're used to being told to dance as if no one is watching, but the reality, especially when we dance in public, is that we're being watched constantly, and this can be a positive thing.

For middle-aged people, I found that dance-confidence levels were much higher in women than in men and that they do not change very much between the late twenties and mid-fifties. One reason for this seems to be that by their mid-twenties, many people have moved on from mate selection and are beginning to settle down with their partner and are starting a family.

However, I also found that many people either change the way they dance or stop dancing altogether once they meet their partner and settle down. This is a relief for some and a frustration for others. While many couples get a huge amount of pleasure from dancing together throughout their lives, some women have complained to me that even though they met their future husband through social dancing (for example at a nightclub), once they settled down he no longer wanted to dance, which in some circumstances stopped her from doing so too.

A man in his early forties said to me:

When I was younger you had to dance either because you were trying to "pull," being told to by your girlfriend, or to show off that you could dance better than your mates. Now I'm older and married the only reason to dance is if the wife nags you. Excuses not to dance are easier now, such as I don't like or don't know the song, my foot's sore or I'm driving (so haven't had a drink). Besides, I prefer to watch the women dance and you can't do that easily if you're dancing and concentrating on your own steps.

And then there was Sofia, a woman in her early fifties who told me about her experience of dancing with another man for the first time after her marriage. Sofia loved to dance. She danced constantly as a child, attending ballet classes every day after school and practicing on a makeshift barre at home. She dreamed of dancing the leading roles on the world's greatest stages. Sofia lived in a small village in eastern Europe and at 15 fell in love with the boy next door. They were married at 17 and she gave birth to her only child, a son, a year later. Her dancing dreams slowly dissolved before they completely disappeared with her marriage to Vladimir and the onset of parenthood. Sofia was now distracted by a different set of daily exercises.

As the years passed, Sofia went back to school, earned several degrees and became a distinguished scientist in the UK. In her university office, she keeps a pair of child's ballet shoes hanging by their ribbons behind her computer. Just before her fiftieth birthday, Sofia decided she wanted to dance again. Her son had grown up and moved on, and Vladimir, a musician, took no interest in dance, so Sofia joined a social-dance class.

Arriving for her first class in nearly 35 years, Sofia was struck by the smell of bodies as she opened the studio door. The room was packed with people finishing an earlier class, and she could taste the atmosphere. Sofia felt heady, and ready to dance. When her class started, she was paired with Robert, an enthusiastic beginner who, she was told, would be her partner for the next ten weeks. Poor Robert, he had no idea what was about to happen. For the first 30 minutes, Sofia and Robert were guided through the basic movements of the cha-cha. Step, step, cha-cha-cha, step, step, cha-cha-cha. Everything was going fine.

The problems started when Sofia and Robert faced one another and got into a Latin hold. She held his left hand with her right, then placed her other hand on his shoulder, while he placed his right hand high on her back. The music started, they made eye contact, and began to dance: Step, step, cha-cha-cha, step, step, cha-cha-cha. They did this four times before Sofia broke hold, turned and ran. She grabbed her bag and her outdoor shoes and she disappeared. Robert was left bewildered. Sofia found her car and cried all the way home.

Vladimir had had an ordinary evening and was watching TV when Sofia came through the front door. She went to the sitting room and told Vladimir that she needed to tell him something. She had stopped crying, but her face was streaked with tears. He thought a terrible thing had happened. As Sofia spoke, the tears came again. She had felt herself falling in love. She had taken Robert in her arms, and he had taken her in his, and as she had looked into his eyes, and as the music had played, and as they danced, she could feel herself falling. The music and the movement had made her forget, for a moment, that she was already in love with, and happily married to, Vladimir. For a moment she was a different person; she had a different life and a different set of dreams. In her yellow dress and suede-soled diamanté-clasped shoes, she saw herself dancing in a grand ballroom and felt what it was like to be carried, and swirled, and swept off her feet. So she had run away.

Vladimir didn't understand. Had she been unfaithful? Was she having an affair? He threw question after question, which she couldn't hear. He saw her experience as an infidelity. He slept in another room and didn't speak to Sofia for ten days. But Sofia hadn't been unfaithful to Vladimir with Robert. And as she lay in their room on her own, she wasn't falling in love with him; she was simply falling back in love with her dreams; she was falling in love with dance and with rekindled feelings.

Vladimir and Sofia are still married. Those old ballet shoes still hang in her office, and Sofia is still afraid to dance.

In older people, I found that dance confidence changed as a function of both sex and age group. In the 56–60 age group, women had higher levels of dance confidence than men, a finding consistent with similar sex differences observed in all younger age groups. However, I also found that for the first time across the lifespan there was no difference between men and women in dance confidence in the over-sixties. At this point, there is a closing of the self-esteem gap because dance confidence drops measurably for women and increases hugely for men.

You might expect, at this age, that there would be a decline in general self-esteem in both sexes, as life begins to take its toll—retirement, loss of life partner, perhaps declining health and lower socioeconomic status. However, if this were the case, then we should expect to see a similar decline in dance confidence in men as well as women.

One of the major life-changing events that happens to women in this stage of life is menopause.

Menopause is the time when estrogen levels fall, there is a change to the menstrual cycle, and eventually, women will stop having periods. Menopause is accompanied by a host of other symptoms, such as hot flushes, night sweats and headaches. The psychological effects can be as heavy as the physical impact. Many women suffer from low moods and anxiety, sometimes for the first time in their life. Some describe the feeling of becoming "invisible," irrelevant, no longer productive and therefore over the hill. No wonder they lose some of their confidence.

Marie told me about her experience with menopause and dancing:

Hot sweats, extreme mood swings, breaking down in a pool of tears and feeling so angry I could seriously do an injury to somebody, and then absolutely calm and back to my old self again. . . . What's all that about? Physically I look in the mirror and I see my Nanna and Mum and a bit of Dad staring back at me, my skin is getting old, I think that I am still like a 30-year-old, but 52 is very different. People see me differently. I went grey/white hair for a bit the other year and realised that people just look through me, almost of no consequence, a sweet older woman. Fuck that, I have dyed my hair brown again with a silver thread at the front and I'm going to grow it long.

Dance has provided me with such a relief from this slow, long road. I meet weekly with a group of women—a great group of women all at different stages in their lives all supporting each other. We do different dance styles and the odd performance. I love it. So far I have done "Shake Your Tail Feather," "All That Jazz" and now we are working on a Madonna routine. I am able to be sassy and best of all have a laugh. I also try to do other dance classes when I can fit it in. In fact, the high I feel after doing a class is probably better than any therapy or medicine anyone can offer, and I am a therapist and I am married to a doctor. It calms my mood, increases my heart rate, gives my brain a break from work and life and I can focus on learning a routine and above all have a laugh. The menopause is something we cannot fight or ignore, we need to accept, understand, acknowledge and move on to enjoy the rest of our lives!

CHOROPHOBIA

There is lack of confidence, and then there is being in a state of full-on terror. In my "Why Do You Dance?"

survey, some respondents expressed a fear of dancing that was heart-breaking to hear. Their fear of dancing was so visceral that it was, in some cases, strong enough to overcome a deep desire and urge to dance. This is a fascinating paradox, rather like being afraid of breathing or eating.

Fear of dancing, also known as chorophobia, is a curious but not uncommon phenomenon. And it can manifest in two ways: as a fear of dancing oneself, and as a fear of seeing other people dance. The major symptoms associated with the former include extreme self-consciousness, avoidance of people and places where dancing happens, social isolation, panic attacks, sweating, nausea, dizziness, heart palpitations, stomach pain and low dance-related self-esteem and confidence levels. The major symptoms associated with the latter include psychological discomfort, distress and aggressive behavior. As with all phobias, these fears are irrational. The act of dancing in and of itself does not pose a threat to anyone's existence, therefore there is no rational reason to be afraid of dancing or watching other people dance. Nevertheless, people's emotional reactions to dance are very real—like an arachnophobe's to spiders—and the distress their fear can cause must not be underestimated.

I have seen all the symptoms of chorophobia over the years. Earlier I described a TV project, where I used dance to help a team of rugby players overcome some of their on-pitch shortcomings. While the whole experience was very productive and positive, there were moments when some of the players showed symptoms of chorophobia. In one session, when I wanted to get them dancing, they became aggressive and evasive; they shouted abuse at me, messed about and caused a lot of disruption. However, when in the next session I reframed the exact same routines as plain and simple movements and exercise, the men behaved with perfect decorum. This type of reaction is the essence of chorophobia.

I love dancing in unusual places and mixing it with activities that are not normally associated with it. This is why I always dance, and encourage the audience to dance, in my lectures. I especially like to experience their emotional reaction to dancing when they are least expecting it. I remember the looks of astonishment on a roomful of Russian bankers in Paris when I started to dance during a talk. They took a while to put down their phones and suspend their disbelief before breaking into dance themselves like proper Cossacks. One of my most memorable experiences was a lecture I gave on the West Coast of the USA. It was amazing surfing the wave of dancing energy that came from the 10,000 business tech-types in the room. But I do not always manage to win people over.

When, in the summer of 2018, I got an email from a scout at a British TV network asking me to take part in a show called *Britain's Got Talent*, I knew it would be a fantastic opportunity to get the world dancing. *Britain's Got Talent* is a talent show judged by the formidable Simon Cowell and the lovely David Walliams, Alesha Dixon and Amanda Holden. It's watched by millions in the UK and has spin-offs around the world.

I agreed to go on the show because I wanted to give the biggest lecture of my life and share my subject with the largest possible audience. Also, I heard that the auditions would be held at the London Palladium, and performing on that stage had been a dream that I never thought would come true. I loved being at the Palladium; I even got to see where Bruce Forsyth's ashes are interred under the stage. In addition, I was keen to experience for myself the emotional roller coaster of auditioning for such a big show. As I walked onto the stage, I felt a bolt of electricity run through my body. Thirty-five years ago, when I was a professional dancer, I used to attend auditions, but they weren't like this.

As I stood center stage facing 3000 audience members and four judges, I felt quite overwhelmed. I told everyone that I was a scientist who wanted to give a lecture about how dancing can be used to improve people's health, well-being and mood. The audience applauded and cheered. As I started my lecture, I asked the audience to stand up, and I quickly taught them a short, fun dance routine and everyone, including all four judges, joined in; even Simon Cowell stood up and wiggled for a moment; I think he even smiled. I told everyone how dancing lifts people's mood and how we have seen this in people with Parkinson's. Then Simon sat down and buzzed, which meant that he wanted the lecture to end. The buzzer was so loud it made the stage vibrate. You don't just hear the buzzer; you feel it too. Although I was expecting to get buzzed—let's face it, I was giving a lecture on *Britain's Got Talent*—when it happened, I didn't know what to do. I thought it was all over and I remember thinking, and perhaps saying out loud, "Oh, should I carry on?" It knocked me off my stride. I did carry on and then I heard a second buzzer, but this was just Simon playing around with David's, so it didn't count.

At the end of the three minutes, I stood and waited for the judges' feedback and their verdict. Simon said he wasn't sure whether there was either too much talking or too much dancing. David, Amanda and Alesha were much more positive. They all gave me a great big yes, and I was told I was through to the next round. Thinking back on the audition after-wards, what I remembered was how flustered Simon had looked, and I think part of that was due to his own dancing, which made him feel uncomfort-able, whereas the other three were very comfortable with letting their bodies move naturally to different rhythms.

Dancing can be scary. I understand that. But re-member the fear is in your head. We were born to dance. You just have to feel the fear and do it anyway.

HAVING THE "WRONG BODY"

I've met lots of people who would be happier to dance in their imaginations and not have to put their body on the line to dance and get groovy. And I under-stand. I have frequently felt at odds with my own body, which is certainly not the perfect body for dance. It used to be better, but even in its prime I thought my legs were two inches too short. Had they been two inches longer, things would have been very different, I'm sure; just two extra inches on each leg would have given me an enormous four inches in toe-to-toe spread as I jumped. It would have transformed my leap. I no longer worry about my two too-few inches. Now I'm worried about excess rather than lack in measurements. When I danced professionally, I was a lithe 126 pounds; now I'm about 210 pounds and I feel like I've gotten shorter too, but perhaps that's just a visual illusion. Dancing with a bigger body presents all kinds of challenges, but they're all just in my head, mostly; my leaps are shorter, obviously, because I'm both older and heavier, and I don't fold from the middle quite so easily. But most of the issues about my dancing body are psychological. I look in the mirror and expect to see a 126-pound frame, and I look around the room and feel as though I stand out because I am heavier than almost everyone else. Of course I stand out. But it really doesn't matter. I know from my research how many other people feel the way I do—it is part of being human, and I do my best not to dwell on these feelings because dancing also makes me feel good.

AGE IS NO OBSTACLE

So much for a lack of dance confidence and an extreme fear of dancing as barriers to entry. Let's now look at some of the other things that stop us from doing it, even when we want to.

Marie, in her description of using dance to beat menopause, shows how dancing can make us feel robust and carefree, and how it can be the ultimate antidote to our fear of aging.

Quite simply, we should all dance our way through our old age, because it not only brings us joy, but it is also a brilliant way to overcome some of the challenges posed by our changing bodies. Dancing has been shown to increase upper-body strength, flexibility, lung capacity and bone mineral content; it can help reduce body mass index (BMI) and heart rate. Scientific studies have also shown that dancing improves balance, walking and bodily awareness and can even reduce people's perception of pain (I guess that's why people can dance the night away in stiletto heels). With all these physical benefits, it is no wonder that dancing is starting to be prescribed by medical doctors, and in some countries people are allowed to spend personal health budgets on certain types of dancing.

The health benefits you will get from different forms of dancing will depend, to a certain extent, on the type of dancing you do. Every form has its own "personality" or set of characteristics. Some forms of dance are social and extroverted, while others are solitary and quiet; some are spontaneous and creative, while others are traditional and rule-based. But one thing is for sure: the more energetic forms of dancing—disco, jazz, tap, fast ballroom, for example—are as good a form of exercise as many track and field sports.

The intensity of different physical activities is measured in units called METs, or metabolic equivalents, on a scale of 1 to 18.[29] For example, resting (sitting quietly in a chair doing nothing) has a MET score of 1, while fast running has a MET of 18. All other physical activities come somewhere in between. So the fast chopping of a tree with an ax has a MET of 17, boxing in a ring has a MET of 12, general bike riding has a MET of 8 and sexual activity has a MET somewhere between 1 and 1.5. To put that into context, engaging in sexual activity uses the same physical intensity as sitting in a chair. I do feel sad for the sexual partners of the scientists who made this decision.

And what of dancing? Well, MET intensity levels for different types of dance range from 2.5 to 10, which means dancing is as intensive as taking part in, say, steeplechase and hurdles, and far better than sex. Added to which, you can dance on your own, with a partner or in a big social group. You can dance with a dozen different people in one evening, and you're not very likely to fall asleep immediately after a three-minute rumba.

MOTIVATION—THE WHY OF BEHAVIOR

Ah yes, motivation. Or lack of it. Of all the reasons people find not to dance, this is one of the most intractable. People often know all about the health benefits of dancing and they know that they "should" be dancing, they even "want" to dance, but they seem to have lost their motivation down the back of the sofa.

I'm writing this on an airplane as I head from London to Orlando for a conference. On the way to the airport, two of my trains were canceled and I had to get a long-distance taxi to arrive on time. Simon was the taxi driver, and we got chatting about movement and exercise. He told me that being a professional driver, first of trucks, then buses and now of taxis, had been bad for his health, because he sat down all day. He told me that he wanted to move more and had often thought of dancing as a way of combining exercise with a social activity so that he could spend more time with his wife. But he got so tired driving all day that all he did when he got home was sit down, again, and watch TV. He then told me why he needed to move more. His dad, who was in his mid-eighties, had just had a major heart attack. Simon recognized that his own lifestyle might be contributing to an increased risk of him having one as well. He said he felt overweight, that he got out of breath when walking upstairs and ate lots of fast food. He was scared of having a heart attack and wanted to do as much as he possibly could to prevent one. He had all the relevant information, he knew his lifestyle was bad for him and he'd had a glimpse into what the future might hold. Nevertheless, despite knowing all this, he was still choosing not to move. His end-of-the-day tiredness, which he knew was caused by his sedentary lifestyle, prevented him from changing his potentially life-threatening routine.

So what do we know about motivation, and how can we use this to help become more active through dance? One of the major problems with traditional forms of exercise is that people start with good intentions but quickly drop out.

A few years ago, the UK consumer organization Which? published the findings of research on its website that suggested that people in the UK are wasting about £37,000,000 ($46.7 million) per year on unused gym memberships.[30] Yes, 37 million pounds every year! People are clearly motivated to join a gym and attend regularly at first because they know it will be good for them, but despite buying all the gear, they soon stop attending. Nevertheless, they continue to pay the monthly fees, presumably because they intend to return.

A fabulous study carried out in Greece looked at the motivation to exercise of middle-aged men with chronic heart failure.[31] The men were divided randomly into three groups. One group had to do lots of Greek dancing, the second one had to do lots of gym-based exercise and the other one didn't have to do anything, apart from their normal day-to-day activities over a period of eight months. Their hearts and physical well-being were tested at the beginning and again at the end of the study. When the results were published, three amazing things were seen.

Firstly, attrition rates were much higher in the gym-based exercise group than in the Greek dance group. In other words, men assigned to the gym-based exercise group got bored and eventually stopped going to the gym, whereas the men assigned to the Greek dancing group clearly enjoyed the experience and kept dancing until the end of the eight-month trial.

Here's the thing: there are two types of motivation, extrinsic motivation and intrinsic motivation. Extrinsic motivation is where you are motivated to do something because somebody has told you you *have* to do it, or because you feel you owe it to someone else to do it. Intrinsic motivation, on the other hand, is all about your subjective experiences of doing something. In other words, you are doing something because you *want* to do it, not because someone else is putting pressure on you. Intrinsic motivation is about doing something for enjoyment or because you are interested in it, or because you think it is important that you do it. In this study there was a huge difference in intrinsic motivation between the men in the Greek dancing group and the men in the gym-based exercise group: the men in the Greek dancing group said that they danced because they enjoyed it, and they felt it was doing them good. The men in the gym-based exercise group, on the other hand, were less intrinsically motivated: they said they enjoyed it less and got bored, which made them drop out and discontinue with the exercise.

Secondly, after eight months on the study, the men who did the Greek dancing showed huge improvements in cardiovascular functioning, but there were no such improvements in the men in the "do nothing" group. Clearly, dancing for eight months is a fantastic way to help a heart recover, while sitting still for months on end is not. And finally, there was an improvement in the general health of men in both the dance and the exercise groups.

If you want to increase your motivation to dance, you need to turn your extrinsic motivation into intrinsic motivation. Another good way of doing this is to come up with a motivation checklist based on Helpful and Unhelpful Motivations.

Remember, you are in charge of the way you think—it is up to you to keep your head filled with helpful motivations. Go on. You know you're worth it!

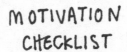

MOTIVATION
CHECKLIST

<u>HELPFUL MOTIVATIONS</u>

- because I enjoy it
- because it is part of who I am
- because I value the benefits of dancing

<u>UNHELPFUL MOTIVATIONS</u>

- because I would feel guilty if I quit
- because people push me to dance, but I question why I continue

CHAPTER 6

THE DANCE CURE

"There is a vitality, a life force, an energy, a quickening that is translated through you into action, and this expression is unique. . . . It is not your business to determine how good it is nor how valuable nor how it compares with other expressions. It is your business to keep it yours clearly and directly, to keep the channel open."

—Martha Graham

Peple have been using dance to enhance health and well-being for hundreds of years. Famously, Captain James Cook, the commander of HMS *Endeavour*, ordered his crew to dance the sailor's hornpipe as they sailed through the Atlantic and the southern Pacific Ocean towards New Zealand and then Australia. HMS *Endeavour* set sail from Plymouth in 1768 on its exploratory expedition. It was at sea for three years. Because the space on board the ship was limited, dancing the "jig of the ship," as Samuel Pepys had referred to it, was thought to be a great way for the sailors to keep fit. They could dance along to music played either on a fiddle or a hornpipe. The basics of this solo dance, which dates back to the fifteenth century, are simple. It involves lots of jumping and hopping on the spot, so gets the heart pumping. As the sailors become more accomplished, they introduce more complex stepping patterns and rhythms, increasing the physical and cognitive challenge of the dance.

Captain Cook knew the key to a successful global voyage of discovery was the good health of his sailors and crew. With the ship thousands of miles from shore, and not knowing for certain when land would be seen again, Cook couldn't risk the negative consequences of a sedentary and unhealthy lifestyle, so he ordered his crew to dance.

He knew a thing or two, did Captain Cook: that dancing keeps us sane and well, and that it should be much more center stage in social and working life.

If I stumbled across Aladdin's lamp and a genie granted me three wishes, here's what I'd wish for. One, I'd wish to change social perceptions so that dancing would be seen to be as normal as walking and drinking coffee. There'd be no taboo about feeling the groove and moving. People would just strut along the street on the way to work or school—dancers alongside joggers and rollerbladers and cyclists.

Two, I'd want Dr. Dance Boogie-Booths constructed in every public space, such as train stations, airports, workplaces, schools, shopping centers, museums and government buildings. Dr. Dance Boogie-Booths are immersive sound-proof rooms where you can dance, literally, as if no one is watching. Some are even big enough for lots of people to dance together. You go into a Dr. Dance Boogie-Booth and lose yourself. They're great for the heart and mind.

And three, I'd wish that free and expressive movement would become a fundamental human right and that the role of movement in enhancing the human experience would be universally recognized. Teachers wouldn't be allowed to tell students off for fidgeting or moving in class, and workplaces wouldn't be allowed to restrict people's movement as they did their jobs. Offices would have fully sprung dance floors rather than carpets. It would be the employees' right to ask at interview how their fundamental right to feel the groove would be honored in the workplace, and it would be enshrined in law that if more than four people were ever standing together in a line or had formed a queue, then they should join together in the queue-dance.

I firmly believe that if dance became an institutionalized part of daily life, we would be a happier, healthier society. But given the unlikelihood of companies encouraging the right to groove any time soon, I must content myself with offering dance prescriptions on an individual level.

One thing I have learned during my decades of dancing and teaching dancing is that, truly, whatever your particular situation or condition, there is a dance or a way of moving your body that can help. And for this chapter, I have had some fun and drawn up ten key dance-based prescriptions to help improve all sorts of aspects of mental and physical health—everything from de-stressing to improving your relationships. There are dances that can be done by individuals and in groups, and by people of different ages and abilities. Just go for the ones that appeal to you.

First, though, a brief word on breathing . . .

NB—If you are in poor health, or recovering from an injury, then you should seek medical advice before engaging in any new physical activity. Once you have been given the all-clear to exercise, you can enjoy all the dances that follow to your heart's content.

BREATHING

We all know how to breathe—it's something we do thousands of times every day without thinking about it. Nevertheless, when we do become aware of our breathing and use it in harmony with our movements, we can transform the way we move and feel.

At a functional level, breathing brings oxygen to our blood, muscles and every cell in our body. With each inhalation of breath, our lungs inflate, our rib cage expands and our diaphragm contracts downwards, and on every exhalation, our body performs the reverse sequence and we rid ourselves of carbon dioxide.

The world's best dancers use breath control as a central part of their training and performance, and we can all apply the same techniques to add effect to our own movements. Here are the four most important lessons I have learned from working closely with professional dancers.

1. Use your breath to control your emotions

To dance and move with purpose, we need to have maximum control of our muscles, but this can be very difficult if they are in a state of immovable tension. Stress and anxiety can lead to a tightening of

the muscles and shallow breathing, but we can re-
lieve some of that stress by focusing on our breathing
and taking control of it. Follow this simple exercise:
take a deep breath . . . and slowly exhale. Again. Be
conscious of your body posture: lower your shoulders, stand centered on your core, take another deep
breath . . .

2. Use your breath to control your expressiveness

For maximum expressiveness, we need to synchronize our movements with our breathing. In ballet
we often start our warm-ups with a series of *pliés*, an
exercise that consists of standing at the barre, bend-
ing our knees and then straightening them. This is a
great place to start to think about pairing our breath
with our movement. Hold on to something at just
about waist height—for example, the back of a chair.
Breathe in, then as you bend your knees, breathe out,
and try to make the length of the breath the same as
the length of the time it takes to fully bend your legs.
Now breathe in as you straighten your legs and return to full height. You can do the same coordinated
movement and breathing exercise with your arms. It
feels beautiful when you move your arms at the same
rate as your breathing, and suddenly a simple *port de
bras* becomes as expressive as a Wordsworth poem.

If you get the chance to watch a live performance of a classical ballet, such as *Swan Lake*, by a professional company, look out for the ways the dancers use breathing and movement to express their feelings.

3. Use your breath to control your stamina

Dancing can be physically demanding and exhausting. I've written before about how dancers have to make what they do look effortless, while beneath the serene surface their pistons are firing at a furious rate. If they are out of breath, they are also out of control. To regain it, they have to learn how and when to calm their heart rate. The best dancers manage to find moments during busy dance routines when they can slow their breathing down. They take a series of long, slow in-breaths, then hold their breath for a few beats, before slowly exhaling through their mouth while supporting their ribs and diaphragm. Try it. It works.

"Don't forget to breathe" is a phrase I've heard dance teachers say a million times over. Sometimes people concentrate so much on their physical movements that they forget to do it. Breathing and moving go hand in hand, and it is vital that as you think about your moving body you also think about the breaths that give life to those movements.

So here we go: the Dance Cure.

1. THE DANCE CURE PRESCRIPTION FOR PROLONGING YOUR LIFE

Physical activity, such as dancing, can reduce all-cause mortality more effectively than medication. Fact. A study published in the *British Medical Journal* in September 2019 found that regular dancing led to a 20–30% lower risk of depression and dementia, a 30% lower risk of colon cancer, a 20% lower risk of breast cancer and a 20–35% lower risk of cardiovascular disease.[32]

Most of us make space for a medicine cabinet in our home, but how many of us make space for a place to dance? Well, everyone has a place to dance at home because we can do it wherever we are; sitting on the sofa, standing in front of the TV or lying on the bed. If you've got a space to boil an egg, you've got a space to boogie.

If you are new to dance or find it hard to get started, try a "follow-me" dance style that is matched to your physical abilities. There are hundreds to choose from, but Zumba is a great place to start because it's suitable for all ages, fitness levels and dance abilities, plus you don't even have to attend a class: you can dance along at home to an online session.

Zumba is a dance form that gets your heart rate

up; it is danced to party-style music, with the teacher leading the class in a sequence of simple dance routines. Follow-me sessions are fabulous for fitness, they're simple and energetic, and because you'll be dancing to some great tunes, they really do provide the basis for a glitter ball–tastic disco party.

2. THE DANCE CURE PRESCRIPTION FOR INCREASING EMPATHY AND BUILDING BETTER SOCIAL RELATIONSHIPS

How empathetic are you? An empathetic person is someone who can place themselves in another's position and has an understanding of their feelings and experiences. Empathy is a type of emotional intelligence that is fundamental to human relationships, because it helps us create meaningful connections. It enables us to appreciate a situation from someone else's perspective and understand their discomfort or distress. Wayne McGregor, resident choreographer at the Royal Ballet, gave a great example of how dance can promote community cohesion when interviewed by Kirsty Young on *Desert Island Discs*. He described a project he had led in Northern Ireland, where 100 young people across the Protestant and Catholic communities came together to perform a dance in front of their families, in a neutral site. McGregor said that by dancing together, they were able to transcend immediate political tensions, and the experience showed them "something of what cooperation and working together looks like." He put it this way:

> [When you dance], you generate a conversation through a body beyond words. . . . If I'm experiencing somebody's weight when they're falling backwards, I'm responsible for making sure that they don't fall. . . . When you actually feel a body, a real presence in real time, it affects everything about how you feel about that body—it personalises it. It becomes about the individual and you realise that they are made of the same flesh and blood. It tells you more about your similarities than your differences.

As this example demonstrates, dance is a great way of improving your emotional intelligence skills. Studies have shown that people who score higher on tests of emotional intelligence tend to be more successful in life.[33] The great thing is that it is not fixed—you can always work on improving your empathetic skills, and dancing is a great way of doing so.

The Gay Gordons is a Scottish country dance that can offer a window into the souls of those dancing it together. The moves are simple to learn, but it takes some skill and practice to execute with a partner. You hold both your partner's hands and start by walking forward, then turning around and walking backwards, then walking forward again before turning around and walking backwards. Then you turn on the spot, under the arm of your partner, before joining together in a waltz hold and polkaing around the room. The Gay Gordons is a wonderful dance for strengthening emotional-intelligence skills, because you need to understand where your partner is in space and time, to think about where they need to be in a few counts' time and to help them arrive there (all the time keeping track of where you yourself are in space and time). When I watch people dance the Gay Gordons, I can see which dancers are empathetically supporting one another and which are resisting the need to adapt based on the needs of another person. In one class, I had a woman who wouldn't be guided by her husband in the Gay Gordons, but was happy to be guided by another man. Watching her dance with these two men was like watching two completely different women dance, interact and move.

Another dance style to try is contact improvisation. This is an improvised, spontaneous form of movement that is based on touch and physical dialogue—imagine having a conversation with someone in which you substitute words with physical contact. Contact improvisation requires movement empathy because you have to be sensitive to the movements and limitations of the other people you are either moving with or around and adjust your own movements accordingly. It is a fantastic way of developing sensitivity to the weight, force and dynamics of other people's characters and emotional states.

3. THE DANCE CURE PRESCRIPTION FOR DE-STRESSING AND STRENGTHENING RESILIENCE

Everyone feels some level of stress and tension at certain times in their lives. The right amount of stress can be helpful, as it pushes us forward as we prepare for something, such as an exam, but when the level of stress reaches a point where the demands outweigh our resources, we can feel mentally or emotionally overwhelmed. The common physical signs of stress include an increased heart rate, faster breathing, tense muscles and sweating. Prolonged stress can lead to headaches, disturbed sleep and fatigue.

Emotional resilience is our ability to adapt to challenging circumstances, to recover quickly from difficulties and spring back into shape. Like empathy, emotional resilience is not fixed at birth—it is a trait that can be developed, and we can all do things to both maintain and enhance it. We know that we need to connect with others to feel and stay well; we need to be physically active and pay attention to our physical health; and we need to give ourselves a break—by being kind to ourselves, taking time out and using hobbies and interests to relax.

The punk-era pogo is the perfect dance to banish stress and enhance resilience. Punks danced to the music of the Sex Pistols and the Clash in the 1970s by jumping up and down, as though they were bouncing on pogo sticks, and wildly crashing into each other. Dancing in such a way meant they had to develop the ability to recover and adjust quickly to the crowded dance floor—an excellent lesson for learning how to deal with the challenges of life. (For inspiration, try watching the video of Debbie Harry explaining pogo to the American people on YouTube—although she does include some surprising additions to the moves!)

If you don't fancy the frenzy of the pogo, there are other dances that can help you think about resilience. If you are a novice dancer, try the cha-cha, or, if you are more experienced, research and learn one of the following dances: the Chacarera from Argentina, the Carolina Shag from the USA, the Chumak from Ukraine or the Romvong from Thailand. Learning a difficult dance style can be frustrating and stressful, but by breaking it down and working on it over several weeks, you can really develop your emotional-resilience skills.

4. THE DANCE CURE PRESCRIPTION FOR GETTING YOURSELF OUT OF A RUT

We take our personal environment for granted. Thinking differently about the things we do and how we interact with our world on a daily basis challenges us to consider the values we place on aspects of our lives. Always doing and thinking about things in the same way gets us into a rut. Dancing can get us out.

The sailor's hornpipe is a dance performed on board ships, originally used to keep sailors physically active on long voyages. It was choreographed to represent the types of movements carried out at sea. The actions mimicked winching the sails, scrubbing the deck, and looking out to the horizon for land. Taking inspiration from this nautical jig, try thinking about the movements that are typical of *your* world, school or workplace environment. To start with, choose a repetitive jumping or skipping step. Then, think about four actions that represent your daily tasks or things you typically carry out throughout the day—perhaps you sit at a computer and type, or you swing a hammer, or you stock shelves in a supermarket. Think about one of the movements you do over and over again, and then start to mix it up. Perhaps you can do it in super-slow motion. Feel how the movement uses some parts of the body more than others. Once you've done this, embellish the movement. For example, incorporate other parts of your body into it.

Changing the way you interact with your environment and physically perform your daily activities will change the way you think about the habits that create your rut. Imagine it being built from lots of small, individual habits—like bricks in a wall. It's only when you are aware of these habits that you can start to plan and execute your escape. Doing this exercise will help you break down the bricks that confine you, and change the habits, first subtly, then dramatically.

5. THE DANCE CURE PRESCRIPTION FOR LEARNING TO LOVE YOURSELF

As a young teenager, I used to dance myself into a euphoric state. I would play records in my bedroom and dance and dance and dance until my head buzzed.

Nothing else gave me the rush I got from dance. My bedroom window overlooked a busy road. At night, I would open the curtains, turn on the lights and dance in front of the window-turned-mirror for hours at a time. I was completely unaware that everyone outside could see me. I must have looked ridiculous, a sweaty teenage boy bouncing frantically around the room, but I didn't care, because I felt fabulous.

If you have been feeling unsure of yourself, or lacking in self-esteem, dancing privately can be a marvelous way of rekindling some self-love. It enables you to try new moves and experiment. It gives you the space and time to lose yourself in the music and movement, to really get to know yourself, which in turn will help release you from self-consciousness. As you start to feel stronger in private, you will find you are feeling more confident in public too.

Try this experiment, and while you are doing it, think about the difference between your public and private selves. First, lock yourself away in glorious solitude, play your favorite tunes and dance. Whether you dance to Gloria Gaynor singing "I Will Survive," or Gershwin's "Rhapsody in Blue," express the real you, your thoughts and feelings, through your movements. Then, take the essence of your private dance and, in your mind, turn it into a public routine. If you did this, what part of the private dance would you leave in, and what would you leave out? Which bits of the real you would you share, and which bits would you hide? What does this make you think about the differences between the private and the public you?

6. THE DANCE CURE PRESCRIPTION FOR HELPING YOU TO MANAGE CHANGE

We all make transitions as we change and develop. For example, from childhood to adulthood, from junior to senior, from subordinate to boss, from single person to partner—and indeed from partner back to single person. Some of these changes come easily; it's as if we have been ready and waiting for them all our lives, whereas others are difficult and uncomfortable. Two of the most challenging aspects of making transitions are dealing with how other people see and respond to our changed role, and internally recognizing and accepting our new social identity and banishing the idea of "imposter syndrome."

A country line dance is an excellent way to help us think about the changes that happen in our lives—and how to face up to them. Once you have learned the basic movements of a line dance, you repeat them as you face in different directions, front, back, right and left. This confuses a lot of people, because inevitably we get used to doing things with a consistent outlook, and if we change that outlook it can push us out of our comfort zone. Sometimes the sequence of steps can change as we move around the room, just as aspects of ourselves change as we move through life.

7. THE DANCE CURE PRESCRIPTION FOR RESOLVING SOCIAL CONFLICT

Dancing or moving is a great way of releasing the tension of conflict, whether it's having a showdown with your teenager or a full-on corporate boardroom argument. Moving can often release the block and help find the way towards an amicable solution.

For the next seven days, make a note of some examples of competition and conflict that you see in the news, on TV or in real life. Jot down too the movements and gestures the people make during these confrontations. What role does movement play in communicating their behaviors? Then, thinking about the interpersonal conflict you are experiencing, make a list of the movement characteristics that you and the people you are in conflict with are using, such as folding arms defensively, keeping a large physical distance apart, not making eye contact, etc. Now, it's your turn to create a new social dance with these people. You don't need to say anything to them; you just need to change the way you interact with them. For example, don't cross your arms in their company, and try changing your personal space when you're around them (by sitting closer or farther away from them, sitting sideways-on rather than face-to-face, or standing instead of sitting), and increase the amount of eye contact you make with them. You will notice positive changes in lots of areas of interpersonal interaction.

A dance form that is fantastic for curing social conflict is hip-hop. A therapist told me about an anger management group she ran with some young offenders. She introduced a hip-hop dance-off halfway through the session, which had the amazing effect of releasing the tension of talking about gang violence and knife crime. At the core of social conflict is often a simmering silence, unspoken words and resentments. Hip-hop provides an outlet for those deep-rooted thoughts and feelings, through the body and face. The movements of hip-hop are unsanitized; they're improvised, raw and emotive.

Practice in the mirror, projecting the character at the heart of your conflict into the reflection, and saying with your body what you cannot say in a traditional conversation. Once you are confident in your moves, you can even take part in face-to-face dance battles, where you can let it all out. Just take the example of the Passinho dance craze in Brazil, which swept to fame after a group of teenagers posted a video of themselves fooling around during a backyard dance-off. The clip went viral and inspired hundreds of young Brazilians to adopt their moves, breaking down stereotypes of violence and criminality among the *favela* youth and instilling the Passinho so deeply into Brazilian culture that it was chosen for the opening dance of the 2016 Rio Olympics. (Search for "Passinho Foda" to see the video that inspired it all—and if you're feeling really adventurous, try out some of the steps yourself!) Whatever bedroom dance you choose, feel the liberation. It will change the way you interact with people in the real world.

8. THE DANCE CURE PRESCRIPTION FOR DECISION MAKING AND PROBLEM SOLVING

All of us will have experienced at some point in our lives the mental conflict associated with being unable to make a decision or solve a particular problem. I once heard a professor talk about this mental conflict in terms of a thirsty mule. He told the class that if you place a thirsty mule exactly halfway between two buckets of water, it will die of thirst, because it won't be able to make up its mind about which bucket to walk towards.

Most of the day-to-day problems we have to solve are trivial and have little consequence in the big scheme of things: which pair of socks to wear, what to eat for dinner, which movie to watch. However, some problems can have a profound impact on our lives: whether to apply for a certain job, whether to leave an unhappy relationship, whether to go to see the doctor about that annoying lump under your arm. The process of problem solving involves thinking about lots of potential solutions, evaluating each one, then making a decision. In some cases, you many need to review the decision in light of new information and keep open the option of altering the solution as time goes on. Some people, and groups of people, find it almost impossible to solve a problem because they get too bogged down in the decision-making process. We call this "paralysis by analysis."

The prescribed cure here is a group dance activity, in which you are forced to make decisions on the spur of the moment. You'll need some other people to dance with and some music.

- Stand in a circle and hold hands.

- Starting on your left foot, take eight steps to the left (this should take 8 counts), then take eight steps to the right (again, 8 counts).

- All walk into the middle of the circle and clap (this should take 4 counts—you clap on 4) and then walk back to where you started and hold hands (again, 4 counts).

- For the final 8 counts everyone should walk back into the middle, forming the circle again, but this time you must make sure you are standing next to someone different, ready to repeat the moves.

The reason this dance is fabulous for thinking about mental conflict is that you cannot plan exactly where you'll be at every point in the dance because it is contingent on the choices made by other people. Just like in life.

9. THE DANCE CURE PRESCRIPTION FOR ENHANCING CREATIVITY

A key aspect of creativity is being receptive to new ideas, sensations and influences, and being prepared to make changes to what we or others have created before. This process of continuous change and development is known as "creative evolution."

Improvisation is at the core of creative evolution. It is about creating something new, on the spur of the moment, without pre-planning. It might be seen as the opposite of acting based on rational thought. To improvise is to be spontaneous—to be unconstrained and to act in a voluntary way, without concern for a given set of rules or boundaries.

Of course, our freedom sometimes needs to be balanced with our obligations to think and act within certain social rules. One of my favorite examples of this tension between freedom and social rules is that of Stephen Gough, otherwise known as the "naked rambler." By 2015, Gough had spent over eight years in prison for refusing to wear clothes in public. He wasn't a flasher or a sex offender; he just didn't want to wear clothes.

In a dance context, Zadie Smith describes the

difference between rule-based, prescriptive dancing and liberated, care-free dancing using the example of the Nicholas Brothers—two outstandingly talented African American dancers whose performance in the film *Stormy Weather* Fred Astaire called "the greatest example of cinematic dance he ever saw." Smith writes:

> I always think I spot a little difference between Harold and Fayard, and it interests me, I take it as a kind of lesson. Fayard seems to me more concerned with [the] responsibility of representation when he dances: he looks the part, he is the part, his propriety unassailable. He is formal, contained, technically undeniable: a credit to the race. But Harold gives himself over to joy. His hair is his tell: as he dances it loosens itself from the slather of Brylcreem he always put on it, the irrepressible Afro curl springs out, he doesn't even try to brush it back. Between propriety and joy, choose joy.[34]

Look up the video of the Nicholas Brothers in *Stormy Weather* to see the moment Smith is talking about, and I challenge you not to smile.

Experimenting with spontaneous movements without worrying about propriety is a hugely beneficial experience. Contemporary dance is a great way to try this out, as it is inherently creative, and involves moving in novel shapes and patterns. For some people, trying contemporary dance for the first time can feel odd and uncomfortable, because you might be doing things with your body that you have never done before. If that's how you feel, don't fight it—go with it and see where it takes you.

Improvising on the dance floor, experiencing the freedom and spontaneity of moving to your favorite tune, can be a catalyst for letting go of rationality. For this, it has to be disco. Or rock. But here's the thing: you have to mix it up. It's easy to fall into set patterns of movement—step-touch, step-touch, step-touch—which is fine as a starting point, but try to do something else at the same time. Make big movements, small movements, try to move every movable part of your body (not necessarily at the same time) and feel the freedom.

10. THE DANCE CURE PRESCRIPTION FOR IMPROVING SELF-CONFIDENCE AND GENERAL WELL-BEING

Dancing gives us a pulse, a spark of life. It facilitates the ultimate mind–body connection and is a brilliant way of making us feel happier in our skin.

What sort of relationship do you have with your body? Although we live with it from birth to death, it is ever changing. It gets bigger and smaller, bits stop functioning properly and it slows down, and we have to adapt to these changes. This evolution of our body—the way we see it and the way it is seen by others—forms a large part of our personal identity.

I know from experience that coming to terms with our changing body through aging or illness can hugely enhance our quality of life. So, for this final prescription, there are two forms of dance that I would recommend, both of which can be wonderfully effective at increasing both body awareness and body confidence: belly dancing and ballet.

Belly dancing originated in the Middle East, and different styles have developed in Egypt, Turkey and Lebanon. Start off by rolling your abdominal muscles from your rib cage down to your waist and then turning your hips through a figure-eight pattern. Once you have gotten the hang of that, and you have a nice rolling figure eight going, you can really express yourself by making beautiful arm movements at the same time. Because your abdominal muscles and hips form the core of your body, when these move, everything moves.

A ballet barre is a set of ballet exercises generally

carried out while holding on to a barre, or the back of a chair. Ballet is fantastic exercise because it gives almost every group of muscles in the body a stretch, and the rhythm of these muscle movements encourages you to breathe deeply, fully expanding and contracting your lungs. A ballet barre works the whole body with both slow and faster movements. It's the perfect way to spend time thinking about the way your body moves and feels. In my home we have a ballet barre that all the family uses.

CONCLUSION

LET'S DANCE

Dancing, as we have seen, is a gift for body and soul. It cures holistically: as you address one aspect of yourself through dance, you will feel benefits percolate through to your whole being.

Before I end this book, I'd like to offer you some of my favorite definitions and descriptions of the joys of dance by the world's best thinkers and artists, who speak to the universality and diversity of what dancing means.

The American fantasy fiction author Amelia Atwater-Rhodes captures the essence of dance as the intersection between the past and the future, the now: "In a society that worships love, freedom, and beauty, dance is sacred. It is a prayer for the future, a remembrance of the past and a joyful exclamation of thanks for the present."

Dance can certainly be defined as a joyful exclamation of thanks for the present, a celebration that we are here and able to take another breath. Eckhart Tolle, the author of *The Power of Now*, explained it like this: "Life is the dancer and you are the dance."

When I read Tolle's definition, I think of life as being not just our living and breathing self, but rather our connection with both our immediate environment and the universe as a whole. To me, "Life is the dancer" means that the universe is the thing that is dancing, and "you are the dance" means that we, at this moment, are the product, or the result, of the dancing universe.

The extraordinarily expressive dancer Isadora Duncan turned this idea into an almost sacred quest. She wrote: "Dance is the movement of the universe concentrated in an individual."

Isadora's life was full of dance, until her death in 1927, when her long scarf became caught in the wheel of a car she was traveling in. At that moment, the movement of the universe became concentrated in an individual (her), the movement of the car, the wind, the rolling road, the long waving scarf.

Voltaire saw dancing as a more benign activity: "Let us read, and let us dance; these two amusements will never do any harm to the world."

By this I think he meant that both reading and dancing are universally harmonious activities and to engage in them positively is a natural response to being alive. I understand reading, here, in its broadest sense—i.e., not just imbibing the written word, but noticing the movement of the trees, the expression on people's faces and their mood. Dance, too, is a physical and emotional interaction with our environment. It is the heartbeat of social engagement, our connection with the world and the people with whom we live in it.

Dancing makes us happy. It's as simple as that. In Taika Waititi's 2019 film *Jojo Rabbit*, which tells the story of Johannes "Jojo" Betzler, a devoted Hitler Youth member who finds out his mother is hiding a Jewish girl in their attic, there is a wonderful moment when Jojo asks the girl, what is the first thing she will do when she gets her freedom? Her answer is immediate: "Dance."

Thank you for reading to the end of *The Dance Cure*. My farewell message to you is: let's be happier and healthier, let's be more creative, let's be in harmony with the people and things that surround us, and most of all, let's dance.

Remember that whenever you are lost for a little bit of movement or you want to bolster your mood, all you have to do is put on a piece of your favorite music and feel the groove. And if you want one sure-fire winning routine to do this, here is my Dr. Dance Happy Dance (for inspiration, follow the video link at www.peterlovatt.com):

Wave right hand, wave left hand (1–4)

Boogie on down (5–8)

Bow and arrow to the right (1–4)

Click twice to right side, twice to left side (5–8)

Bow and arrow to the left (1–4)

Click twice to left side, twice to right side (5–8)

Rainbow wave from right to left (1–4)

Rainbow wave from left to right (5–8)

Starting on your right foot

Take three steps forward and clap (1–4)

Take three steps backwards and clap (5–8)

Take three steps forward and clap (1–4)

Take three steps backwards and clap (5–8)

Take three steps to the right and clap (1–4)
Take three steps to the left and clap (5–8)
Take three steps to the right and clap (1–4)
Take three steps to the left and clap (5–8)

Step, turn, step to the right and clap (1–4)
Step, turn, step to the left and clap (5–8)
Step, turn, step to the right and clap (1–4)
Step, turn, step to the left and clap (5–8)

Right foot
Heal dig, toe tap, heal dig, toe tap (1–4)
Point right finger across your body and then
    move it from left to right (5–8)

Heal dig, toe tap, heal dig, toe tap (1–4)
Point right finger high to the corner (John
    Travolta–style) then down to your hip, twice
    (5–8)

Heal dig, toe tap, heal dig, toe tap (1–4)
Point right finger across your body and then
    move it from left to right (5–8)

Heal dig, toe tap, heal dig, toe tap (1–4)
Point right finger high to the corner (John
    Travolta–style) then down to your hip, twice
    (5–8)

Now, let your body go and groove to the music. Do whatever feels good, and when you're ready to start the Dr. Dance Happy Dance again, simply put your right hand up in the air, give yourself a 5, 6, 7, 8, and away you go.

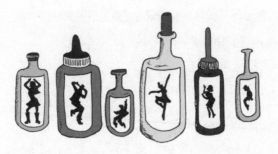

THE DANCE APOTHECARY

This book would not be complete without a full list of remedies from *The Dance Cure* medicine cabinet. So, here are some of my favorite dance tunes, videos and things to turn to when you need inspiration.

DR. DANCE TOP TEN FAVORITE DANCE TUNES

1. MacArthur Park [Suite]—Donna Summer
   (the full 17-minute version)

2. Lost in Music—Sister Sledge
   (1984 Bernard Edwards and Nile Rogers Remix)

3. Rapper's Delight—The Sugarhill Gang
   (12" version)

4. Wham Rap! (Enjoy What You Do?)—Wham!

5. On the Floor—Jennifer Lopez ft. Pitbull

6. Street Life—Crusaders (12" version)

7. Breakin' Down—Julia and Company
   (12" version)

8. Wings (The Alias Radio Mix)—Little Mix

9. Turn the Music Up—The Players Association
   (12" disco)

10. Don't Stop 'Til You Get Enough—
    Michael Jackson (the 6-minute version)

DR. DANCE TOP TEN GROOVY TUNES (SCIENTIFICALLY INSPIRED)

1. Superstition—Stevie Wonder

2. Soul Bossa Nova—Quincy Jones

3. Flash Light—Parliament

4. Sing, Sing, Sing—Benny Goodman

5. In the Mood—Glenn Miller

6. Come Fly with Me—Frank Sinatra

7. Take Five—Dave Brubeck

8. Could You Be Loved—Bob Marley & the Wailers

9. Summertime—Al Jarreau

10. Don't Stop Me Now—Queen

DR. DANCE TOP TEN SHOW TUNES TO SING AND DANCE TO

1. Hello, Dolly!—*Hello, Dolly!* (the original cast recording from the film is my favorite)

2. Good Morning—*Singin' in the Rain* (original cast)

3. Lullaby of Broadway—*42nd Street* (original cast)

4. One—*A Chorus Line* (original cast)

5. Cabaret—*Cabaret* (Liza Minnelli version)

6. Simple Joys—*Pippin* (1972 original cast)

7. America—*West Side Story* (original cast)

8. If I Were a Rich Man—*Fiddler on the Roof* (original cast)

9. Don't Rain on My Parade—*Funny Girl* (the *Glee* cast version is my favorite)

10. I Am What I Am—*La Cage aux Folles* (the George Hearn version is my favorite)

DR. DANCE TOP TEN DANCE SCENES IN MOVIES

1. Moses Supposes—*Singin' in the Rain*
   https://www.youtube.com/watch?v=tciT9bmCMq8

2. What a Feeling—*Flashdance* (1983)
   https://www.youtube.com/watch?v=VzALZjolx0g

3. Rhythm of Life—*Sweet Charity*
   https://www.youtube.com/watch?v=xKSA049xkiU

4. Opening Sequence—*A Chorus Line*
   (1985 movie version)
   https://www.youtube.com/watch?v=EHPdVnUour4

5. Prologue—*West Side Story* (1961)
   https://www.youtube.com/watch?v=bxoC5Oyf_ss

6. Hot Lunch Jam—*Fame* (1980)
   https://www.youtube.com/watch?v=QMMHut0t-HU

7. We're All in This Together—*High School Musical*
   https://www.youtube.com/watch?v=DykVJl6wr_4

8. Heaven—*Top Hat* (1935)
   https://www.youtube.com/watch?v=ILxo-TUkzOQ

9. Shake a Tail Feather—*The Blues Brothers* (1980)
   https://www.youtube.com/watch?v=qdbrlrFxas0

10. The Broadway Melody Ballet—*Singin' in the Rain* (1952)
    https://www.youtube.com/watch?v=QOxpnWbzOco

DR. DANCE TOP TWENTY QUICK DANCE FIXES

1. To feel graceful and proud—try ballet

2. To feel earthy and rhythmic—try tap

3. To feel your pulse and heartbeat—try jazz

4. To feel intellectual—try contemporary

5. To feel in the mood for a party—try Zumba

6. To feel fully alive—try disco

7. To feel young and urban—try street

8. To feel retro and trendy—try lindy

9. To feel spontaneous and competitive—try hip-hop

10. To feel ordered and united—try line dancing

11. To feel confident in your body—try belly dancing

12. To feel expressive yet controlled—try flamenco

13. To feel traditional and rooted —try folk

14. To feel up-close and personal—try Argentine tango

15. To feel strong—try pole dancing

16. To feel cheeky—try burlesque

17. To feel motivational—try cheerleading

18. To feel emotional—try musical theatre

19. To feel sexy—try rumba

20. To feel socially connected—try ceilidh

REFERENCES

1. Winkler, I., Haden, G. P., Ladinig, O., Sziller, I. & Honing, H. (2009). Newborn infants detect the beat in music. *Proceedings of the National Academy of Sciences*, 106(7), 2468–2471.

2. Janata, P., Tomic, S. T. & Haberman, J. M. (2012). Sensorimotor coupling in music and the psychology of the groove. *Journal of Experimental Psychology*: General, 141(1), 54–75.

3. Wang, T. (2015). A hypothesis on the biological origins and social evolution of music and dance. *Frontiers in Neuroscience*, 9(30). doi: 10.3389/fnins.2015.00030.

4. Dunbar, R. I. M. (2012a). Bridging the bonding gap: the transition from primates to humans. *Philosophical Transactions of the Royal Society* B: Biological Sciences, 367, 1837–1846. doi: 10.1098/rstb.2011.0217.

5. Dunbar, R. I. M. (2012b). On the evolutionary function of song and dance, in *Music, Language and Human Evolution*, eds N. Bannan and S. Mithen (Oxford: Oxford University Press), 201–214.

6. Tarr, B., Launay, J. & Dunbar, R. I. M. (2014). Music and social bonding: "self-other" merging and neurohormonal mechanisms. *Frontiers in Psychology*, 5, 1096.

7. Tarr, B., Launay, J. & Dunbar, R. I. M. (2016). Silent disco: dancing in synchrony leads to elevated pain thresholds and social closeness. *Evolution and Human Behavior*, September; 37(5): 343–349. doi: 10.1016/j.evolhumbehav.2016.02.004.

8. Miller, G., Tybur, J. M. & Jordan, B. D. (2007). Ovulatory cycle effects on tip earnings by lap dancers: economic evidence for human estrus? *Evolution and Human Biology*, 28, 375–381.

9. Waller, J. (2009). *The Dancing Plague: The Strange, True Story of an Extraordinary Illness* (Naperville, IL: Sourcebooks, Inc.).

10. Brown, A., Martinez, M. J. & Parsons, L. M. (2006). The neural basis of human dance. *Cerebral Cortex*, 16(8), 1157–1167. https://doi.org/10.1093/cercor/bhj057.

11. Blanchette, D. M., Ramocki, S. P., O'del, J. N. & Casey, M. S. (2005). Aerobic exercise and creative potential: immediate and residual effects. *Creativity Research Journal*, 17(2/3), 257–264.

12. Steinberg, H., Sykes, E. A., Moss, T., Lowery, S., LeBoutillier, N. & Dewey, A. (1997). Exercise enhances creativity independently of mood. *British Journal of Sports Medicine*, 31, 240–245.

13. The TV show was called *Why Don't You?* It was on the BBC from 1973 to 1995. It had a catchy theme tune which went . . . https://www.you tube.com/watch?v=_uvev7hY5MU.

14. Lewis, C. (2012). The relationship between improvisation and cognition. University of Hertfordshire. https://uhra.herts.ac.uk/bitstream /handle/2299/8890/05107372%20Lewis%20Carine%20-%20final%20 PhD%20submission.pdf?sequence=1.

See also: Lewis, C. & Lovatt, P. J. (2013). Breaking away from set patterns of thinking: improvisation and divergent thinking. *Thinking Skills and Creativity*, 9, 46–58.

15. Warburton, E. C., Wilson, M., Lynch, M. & Cuykendall, S. (2013). The cognitive benefits of movement reduction: evidence from dance marking. *Psychological Science*, 24(9), 1732–1739.

16. Walker, M. P., Brakefield, T., Morgan, A., Hobson, J. A. & Stickgold, R. (2002). Practice with sleep makes perfect: sleep-dependent motor skill learning. *Neuron*, 35, 205–211.

17. Hackney, M. E., Kantorovitch, S., Levin, R. & Earhart, G. M. (2007). Effects of tango on functional mobility in Parkinson's disease: a preliminary study. *Journal of Neurologic Physical Therapy*, 31, 173–179.

18. Lewis, C., Annett, L. E., Davenport, S., Hall, A. & Lovatt, P. (2016). Mood changes following social dance sessions in people with Parkinson's disease. *Journal of Health Psychology*, 21(4), 483–492.

19. Livingston, C. & Borko, H. (1990). High school mathematics review lessons: expert-novice distinctions. *Journal for Research in Mathematics Education*, 21(5), 372–387.

20. Carney, D. R., Cuddy, A. J. C. & Yap, A. J. (2010). Power posing: brief nonverbal displays affect neuroendocrine levels and risk tolerance. *Psychological Science*, 21, 1363.

21. Leung, A. K-Y., Kim, S., Polman, E., Ong, L. S., Qiu, L., Goncalo, J. A. & Sanchez-Burks, J. (2012). Embodied metaphors and creative "acts." *Psychological Science*, 23(5), 502–509.

22. Koch, S. C., Morlinghaus, K. & Fuchs, T. (2007). The joy dance: specific effects of a single dance intervention on psychiatric patients with depression. *The Arts in Psychotherapy*, 24, 340–349.

23. Jeong, Y-J., Hong, S-C., Lee, M. S., Park, M-C., Kim, Y-K. & Suh C-M. (2005). Dance movement therapy improves emotional responses and modulates neurohormones in adolescents with mild depression. *International Journal of Neuroscience*, 115(12), 1711–1720.

24. Lane, A. & Lovejoy, D. J. (2001). The effects of exercise on mood change: the moderating effect of depressed mood. *Journal of Sports Medicine and Physical Fitness*, 41(4), 539–545.

25. Health Development Agency (2000). Arts for health: a review of good practice in community-based arts projects and initiatives which impact on health and wellbeing. ISBN: 1-84279-016-1. Retrieved from www.hda-online.org.uk.

26. Burgess, G., Grogan, S. & Burwitz, L. (2006). Effects of a 6-week aerobic dance intervention on body image and physical self-perceptions in adolescent girls. *Body Image*, 3(1), 57–66.

27. Karouda, Y., Geisler, G., Morel, P. C. H. & Hapeta, J. (2017). Stress, emotions, and motivational states among traditional dancers in New Zealand and Japan. *Psychological Reports*, 120(5), 895–913.

28. Lovatt, P. J. (2011). Dance confidence, age and gender. *Personality and Individual Differences*, 50, 668–672.

29. Ainsworth, B. E., Haskell, W. L., Whitt, M. C., Irwin, M. L., Swartz, A. M., Strath, S. J., O'Brien, W. L., Bassett, D. R. Jr., Schmitz, K. H., Emplaincourt, P. O., Jacobs, D. R. Jr. & Leon, A. S. (2000). Compendium of physical activities: an update of activity codes and MET intensities. *Medicine and Science in Sports and Exercise*, 32(9), S498–504.

30. Steen, P. (2011). Are you wasting cash on an unused gym membership? *Which?* https://conversation.which.co.uk/travel-leisure/are-you-wasting-money-on-an-unused-gym-membership/.

31. Kaltsatou, A. C. H., Kouidi, E. I., Anifanti, M. A., Douka, S. I. & Deligiannis, A. P. (2014). Functional and psychosocial effects of either a traditional dancing or a formal exercising training program in patients with chronic heart failure: a comparative randomized controlled study. *Clinical Rehabilitation*, 28(2), 128–138.

32. Haseler, C., Crooke, R. & Haseler, T. (2019). Promoting physical activity to patients. *British Medical Journal*, 366, l5230. doi: 10.1136/bmj.l5230.

33. Chong, S. C., Falahat, M. & Lee, Y. S. (2020). Emotional intelligence and job performance of academicians in Malaysia. *International Journal of Higher Education*, 19(1), 69–80.

34. Smith, Z. (2016). Dance lessons for writers. *Guardian*. https://www.theguardian.com/books/2016/oct/29/zadie-smith-what-beyonce-taught-me.

ACKNOWLEDGMENTS

This book has come to life because of the ideas, energy and creative talents of several people. I would like to start by acknowledging, and thanking, my literary agent, Charlotte Robertson, for her amazing memory, support and encouragement. Charlotte and I first chatted about the ideas in this book several years ago, before we each followed different paths. When our paths crossed again, in early 2019, Charlotte remembered very clearly the feelings I wanted to express in a book about dance, and she helped me to express those feelings in words and she took the ideas to Short Books, which was a perfect fit. I would like to thank my publishers, Aurea Carpenter and Rebecca Nicolson, from Short Books, for commissioning the title and for editing and taming my excessive flow of words. You have them to thank for the linguistic topiary; I would have given you a shaggy bush. I would like to thank Helena Sutcliffe for the wonderful illustrations, which perfectly lift the words from the page, and gives them a dancer's breath.

It is, perhaps, impossible to identify the precise moment an idea is created, or even in whose head. I doubt that I have ever had any good ideas that sprung entirely from my own head. I would like to acknowledge my thinking partner, Lindsey Lovatt. Lindsey and I chat about everything. We play with ideas, we share them, move them, turning them first into one thing, and then another. We tease ideas from each other. All of the ideas in this book have spent as much time whirling around in Lindsey's head as they have in mine.

I feel extremely lucky to have worked with both a thinking partner to shape the ideas and an editorial team to shape the prose. The strength of the book comes from these interactions. Any weaknesses are entirely my own.

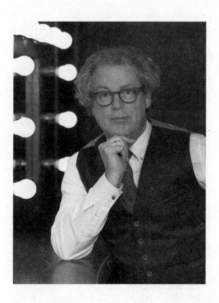

Dr. Peter Lovatt is a dance psychologist. After working as a professional dancer in musical theatre, and overcoming a severe reading difficulty, he took degrees in psychology, English and neural computation, combining a fascination with psychology and neuroscience with his passion for dance. After 15 years of working as an academic, he set up the first Dance Psychology Lab in 2008, where he studied how movement affects social interactions, changes the way people think and solve problems, and enhances human experience. Peter is a popular motivational speaker, inspiring audiences around the world to embrace the transformative power of dance. He is currently delivering a series of lectures on dance psychology at the Royal Ballet School.